What's Stopping You?

What's Stopping You?

Living Successfully with Disability

Mark Nagler, Ph.D.
and Adam Nagler

Published in 1999 by Stoddart Publishing Co. Limited
34 Lesmill Road, Toronto, Canada M3B 2T6

Distributed in Canada by General Distribution Services Limited
325 Humber College Blvd., Toronto, Ontario M9W 7C3
Tel. (416) 213-1919   Fax (416) 213-1917
Email Customer.Service@ccmailgw.genpub.com

Distributed in the U.S. by General Distribution Services Inc.
85 River Rock Drive, Suite 202, Buffalo, New York 14207
Toll-free tel. 1-800-805-1083 Toll-free fax 1-800-481-6207
Email gdsinc@genpub.com

03 02 01 00 99 1 2 3 4 5

Canadian Cataloguing in Publication Data

Nagler, Mark
What's stopping you?: living successfully with disability

ISBN 0-7737-6027-X

I. Handicapped.   I. Nagler, Adam.   II. Title.

HV1568.N33 1999   362.4
C98-933023-0

Cover design: Angel Guerra
Design and typesetting: Kinetics Design & Illustration

Printed and bound in Canada

Stoddart Publishing gratefully acknowledges the Canada Council for the Arts and the Ontario Arts Council for their support of its publishing program.

In memory of Eric Chodak,
who showed us all how to live with a disability

Contents

Acknowledgments

Many people helped us write this book. First, we would like to thank our family, who has been wonderfully supportive throughout this entire project. We could not have written this book without David, Sharon, and Mother. Ernie and Janie Nagler also provided comments and stories for us. Indeed, everyone who inspired the case studies in this book has earned our appreciation for their courage.

Our colleagues have been very supportive, particularly the faculty of Renison College and the University of Waterloo. Karen McCallum, Jodi Morris, Ruth Ambros, and Monica Walker-Bolton have been most helpful. Thanks to Craig McFadyen and the Ontario Ministry of Intergovernmental Affairs for showing great flexibility when deadlines loomed.

Larry Hoffman's insightful comments and encouragement were essential throughout this project. Stoddart Publishing has been very generous in providing time and first-rate personnel.

The astute observations of our editors, Jim Gifford and Donald Bastian, have enriched this work.

Ellard McBane, Michael Peters, Nicholas Brown, and Jack Krieger were most generous in sharing their insurance and investment expertise, and the legal insights provided by Barry Seltzer, David Baker, Kim Carpenter-Gunn, and Rhona Waxman were essential to the sections on law. Lynda Silver-Dranoff's book *Everybody's Guide to the Law* was a fantastic resource for our work on powers of attorney and other aspects of the law. Dr. Bryan Alton provided excellent comments on the manuscript from a medical perspective. Thanks to Mike D'Abramo, Jacob Glick, and Jane Motz for sharing their expertise on computers and Web sites, and to all of the students who helped research this book. Merci, Max Valiquette. Vraiment. Thanks again to our title wizard, Mel Enkin.

Rarely does a father have the opportunity to work with a son who is also a genuine colleague. Adam's penetrating analyses and insights have made this text an accurate representation of what it means to plan for the effects of a disability.

Preparation of *What's Stopping You?* was supported in part by a grant from the University of Waterloo, Social Sciences and Humanities Grant Fund (UW/SSHRC).

Introduction

Overcoming Disability

HOW WE SEE DISABILITY

What images do the word "disability" bring to mind? A pianist playing to sold-out concert houses around the world? A director and movie star raising millions of dollars for charities? A world-renowned physicist? A star pitcher throwing a no-hitter? The president of the United States inspiring his nation? These may not be the roles that most of us would associate with people who have disabilities, but they are accurate and real.

David Helfgott is a classical pianist from Australia who has played to packed concert halls around the world, but who for many years could not even play in public because of mental illness. His story was dramatized in the movie *Shine*. Christopher Reeve, the star of the Superman movies, has overcome quadriplegia to direct and star in a remake of the Alfred Hitchcock thriller *Rear Window* and to raise millions of dollars for spinal-cord research. Stephen Hawking, the author of *A Brief History of Time* is recognized as a leading theoretical physicist. He strongly believes that his battle with amyotrophic lateral sclerosis (also known as Lou Gehrig's disease) has not hindered his career. Jim Abbott, who was born with only one hand, has had a very successful career playing baseball in the major leagues. He even threw a no-hitter while pitching for the New York Yankees. President Franklin Delano Roosevelt overcame polio to serve an unprecedented three straight terms as president and lead the United States to victory in the Second World War.

Each of these people represents a triumph of the human spirit over physical and psychological challenges. They show that disability doesn't have to be limiting; it can open up any number of new opportunities and horizons. These examples are celebrities, but their accomplishments are duplicated every day by "average citizens" whose lives serve as testaments to hard work, independence, and dignity. There are millions of people who live successfully with their disabilities, and who make valuable contributions to the economic, scientific, and cultural fabric of our society. These successes do not come easily, however. It takes courage, insight, perseverance, commitment, planning, and the support of caregivers to surmount the obstacles that disability can create.

Over the course of this book, we will share with you the inspirational stories of some "average people" with disabilities who have overcome many of the same challenges you may encounter.[1] Their successes show that you do not have to be wealthy or famous or a genius to overcome disabling conditions.

---

1 The stories and case studies in this book are real, but we have altered names and locations to protect the privacy of those involved.

THE IMPACT OF DISABILITY

How many people do you know who have had to contend with disabilities? How many of your friends or acquaintances have been unable to work for several months or years because of illness or accident? Have you known anyone who has had an extended stay in the hospital, followed by extensive rehabilitation? Have you or anyone you know assumed responsibility for the care of a loved one? If you reflect, you probably know many more people in these categories than you imagined.

How many of the people you know had to start dealing with disability suddenly? Were any of them overwhelmed? Did they take a long time to adjust? If a serious accident happened today that prevented you from working for several weeks, months, or years, would you be ready? If a loved one was seriously injured, would you know how to provide care? Disability can force you to contend with a wide range of issues, including medical care; renovations to the home; a temporary or permanent inability to work, or a need to change occupations; changes to your family; changes to your personal identity; financial pressures; finding new activities; and adapting your personal life to your new physical and psychological reality. With disability, everyone has to cope with these changes. The odds are that someone in your immediate family will have to contend with a serious disability before the age of sixty-five.

Disability is on the rise in our society, but few people want to consider that it might one day affect them. Few people want to discuss the impact of disability on their lives, or to imagine that they might experience an illness or accident, or may have to take care of a parent, child, or spouse with a disability. We are writing this book because we feel that everyone who has a disability, and everyone who will encounter disability, must be made aware of the resources and strategies that can help overcome the challenges that disability poses.

There are more than 58 million people in the United States and Canada living with a disability! The chances of encountering a disability during your lifetime are astronomical. Hopefully, you are healthy and will not face a disability in the near future. Every year, however, hundreds of thousands of people are affected by serious illnesses such as cancer, diabetes, and Alzheimer's disease. Over the course of a lifetime, one in four North Americans will suffer a heart attack or stroke. One in three will develop a life-threatening cancer. One in four will experience kidney disease. Millions more will encounter other disabilities through illness or accident.

Although the elderly are more vulnerable, disability can strike adults of all ages. One-third of stroke victims are under the age of sixty-five, and one-third of those who develop cancer are under the age of forty. These conditions are rarely immediately fatal — the death rate for heart disease has decreased 50 percent in the last thirty years, for example, and the success rate for kidney transplants has reached 85 percent. With these and other improvements in medical technology, more people are living longer than ever with disabilities.

Everyone hopes that if they suffer a serious injury or disease, they will be able to recover quickly and get back to living life just the way they used to. Unfortunately, however, disabilities can bring about drastic changes in lifestyle and affect quality of life. Some people may have to learn how to use a wheelchair, and others may become dependent on caregivers to perform tasks that they once considered routine. Many people will also have to become caregivers for their loved ones. It is difficult to face up to this possibility, but it must be done. You must ask yourself if you have prepared for the consequences of disability, so that you and your family will be protected.

My Story

In early February 1996, I woke up in the morning with severe chest pains, which I thought was just a bad case of heartburn. I called my family physician, and he told me to go directly to the hospital. I arrived at the emergency room, explained my situation, and was immediately hooked up to a heart monitor. I watched my own heart attack occur on the screen! Strangely enough, it was not very painful. The physician explained that I was experiencing a myocardial infarction, which is the medical term for a heart attack. Although I expected to die at any second, I somehow maintained my sense of humour and thanked the doctor for making my day. Within minutes of the heart attack, I had been wheeled into a private room and given a dose of streptokinase, a drug used to minimize the damage to my heart.

After my condition stabilized, I went to sleep, then was confined to bed for several days. I was informed that because I had reached the hospital so quickly, the damage to my heart was minimal. I spent the next week and a half in the hospital, and then I was sent home. During my time at home, I felt very weak and experienced a lot of angina, the chest pain that often follows a heart attack. Five weeks later I had a bout of severe nausea and returned to the hospital. After two days of testing, they determined that I had had a second heart attack. After being in the hospital for three more long weeks, I was finally given an angiogram, which determined that two of my main arteries were completely blocked, and that the only viable treatment would be double-bypass surgery.

I stayed in the hospital until my surgery, which was scheduled for April 25. The surgery was successful, and five days later I was released. After only four days, I was forced to return to the hospital by ambulance. I was suffering from severe breathing problems, pneumonia, a collapsed lung, and an abscessed tooth.

Two weeks later, I was released again. Initially, I was extremely weak. I lost thirty-five pounds (which was not necessarily a bad thing) and had a great deal of difficulty eating. I had to deal with questions about my mortality, my family, my job, my quality of life, and the limitations and other challenges I would have to face. In addition to my questions about the unknown, I also had to deal with physical pain, mental weakness, and depression. Although I have lived my entire life with a disability, coping with the sudden onset of another one was a completely different experience. I had to use all of the skills that I had developed over a lifetime of living with cerebral palsy, as well as learn some new ones.

Following the heart attacks, I had to stop teaching at the university. I was unable to continue serving on a government committee reviewing college administration, and I had to cease my volunteer work. My university had a very generous leave plan, which paid me 100 percent of my wages for the time I was off work. I was fortunate to have been protected by such a generous work-related plan. I gradually regained my strength, and by the following September I was able to resume my teaching obligations.

Since then, I have continued to attend cardiac-rehabilitation classes, watch my diet, and exercise diligently. With my son Adam, I wrote a book entitled *Yes You Can!*, a parent's guide to raising children with disabilities, and have made numerous presentations at academic conferences and conventions.

It has been a constant struggle to overcome my heart attacks, but with the love and support of my family and friends, the aid of the wonderful professionals who helped me plan and achieve my rehabilitation, and my own determination, I have been able to get on with my life. I have made significant changes to my lifestyle, but I am able to maintain a very high quality of life, and I have a deeper appreciation of every day.

My personal experience, my professional work on disability and rehabilitation, and my volunteer work on behalf of people with disabilities provided me with the expertise to write this book. Although I was born with cerebral palsy, which hampers my motor co-ordination, and I have never been able to write, I have earned a B.A., an M.A., and a Ph.D., and have worked as a university professor for thirty years. But despite my background — fifty-nine years of living with a disability, and years of research and activism in the field of disability — I was still not prepared for my heart attack. I just wasn't ready for all changes I had to make. I decided to write this book to help people cope with the challenges that disability may pose — for family members, caregivers, and most important, the individual with the disability.

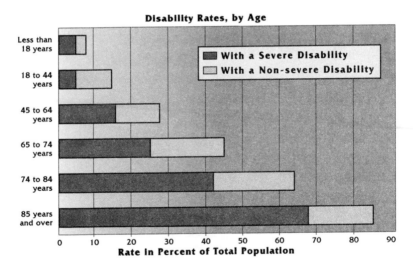

Disability Rates, by Age

With a Severe Disability
With a Non-severe Disability

Less than 18 years
18 to 44 years
45 to 64 years
65 to 74 years
74 to 84 years
85 years and over

0   10   20   30   40   50   60   70   80   90
Rate in Percent of Total Population

PERSONAL ATTITUDES TOWARDS DISABILITY

Most people are optimists and choose not to consider the possibility that they may not always be in perfect health. Disability is something most people are reluctant to think about. "I don't want to hear about it." "It can't happen to me." "It's a waste of time." These are the most common reactions I encounter when I try to discuss the implications of disability with healthy people. Too often, people try to avoid thinking negative thoughts. To others, negative thoughts simply never occur. Too many people are highly vulnerable because they are unable or unwilling to make critically important plans for their future. If you spend some time on self-education, you can save yourself a lot of heartache. Planning is the best way to prevent financial stress or ruin, family stresses, and the other hardships that can accompany disability.

Disability used to be something that society tried to ignore. People with disabilities were placed in institutions, schools and workplaces were inaccessible, and the opportunities for participation and integration were almost non-existent. Because people with disabilities were hidden from view, decision-makers did not have to address their concerns. The status of the "handicapped"[2] community has undergone a dramatic transformation over the last three decades, however. People with disabilities are gaining prominence in many occupations and professions, and the stereotypes are constantly being eroded. This trend will only continue, because the technology that is available to help people with disabilities integrate and rehabilitate is constantly improving. Although we are more likely than ever before to encounter disability, the opportunities to maintain a high quality of life in spite of disability have never been better.

---

2   In our thesaurus, the synonyms for someone with a disability include: "incapacitated, crippled, lame, helpless, impotent, incapable, unable, done for, ineffectual, fruitless, futile, and useless." We do not use any of these terms to describe disability in our book.

   Words such as "crippled," "retarded," "invalid," and "lame" perpetuate inaccurate stereotypes of people with disabilities. They are outdated terms that are no longer relevant in an intelligent discussion of disability. Throughout this book, we use terminology that is "disability-friendly" and does not build on such negative stereotypes.

RESOURCES FOR ACTION

This book will make you aware of the nature and impact of disability, and will help you develop the skills and strategies that are necessary both to contend with a disability and to provide care for a loved one with a disability. In addition to these techniques, we also provide a guide to the different types of disability insurance, and explain how to construct a financial plan that will protect you from the consequences of disability. *What's Stopping You?* will teach you how to become an informed consumer who is able to choose the appropriate personnel, protection, and patterns of care.

We have included a variety of resources that you can use to plan for and cope with disability. These include:

1. A catalogue of sample letters requesting a wide range of information and services, which can be adapted to your individual needs (Appendix A).
2. A directory of North American resource centres and support groups for people with disabilities, which provide up-to-date information on specific disabilities and access to a wide range of help (Appendix B).
3. A bibliography of up-to-date literature on specific disabilities and a list of some of the most important health-related Web sites.

These will direct you to sources of support and information on a wide range of specific conditions. They will help you to follow up on the basic principles that you learn from this book. The right attitude and the wide range of resources that we identify will help you to prepare for and cope with disability.

THE IMPORTANCE OF PLANNING

The majority of people plan for the important events in their lives. Most of us plan for our health care, the education of our children, and our retirement. We plan our careers, our investments, our mortgages, and even our leisure time. Sometimes we do it on our own, and other times we engage professional help. We plan for virtually everything that is important! The one thing that people do not usually plan for, either because they do not know that it's necessary or because they do not want to think about it, is disability. Preparing yourself to deal with a disability, whether it is your own, your spouse's, or your parent's, can be a daunting task. With the proper foresight, however, a potentially devastating situation can be averted.

The theme of planning will run throughout this book. It lays the foundation for your personal approach to disability, for obtaining the best medical and rehabilitative care, for gaining access to support groups and resources, and for helping your family and dependents cope with what can be a tremendous challenge.

THE SANDWICH GENERATION

You may belong to the Baby Boom Generation, and feel that you are still a long way from disability. However, your parents may already be in, or rapidly approaching, "old age." The number of North Americans who are members of the so-called Sandwich Generation is constantly increasing. The people in this group are sandwiched between responsibility for their children and for their parents, in-laws, relatives, and even friends. This responsibility can be financial (paying for or subsidizing residential or home care), custodial (providing care in your home), or emotional (providing needed love and support). For people in this situation, this book contains a chapter on dealing with a parent's disability. Caring for parents who have health problems is hard enough when you are healthy. If you experience a disability during this time, it may be difficult to maintain your role as chief caregiver. We provide the strategies to help you weather this storm.

WHO THIS BOOK IS FOR

This book is a guide to disability for the general public. It is meant to inform you about disability and alert you to the challenges it can pose. This book is also written for anyone who has a disability and is looking for strategies to manage and cope with their condition. Because disability can prevent people from doing things on their own, this book is directed to family members and others who are responsible for the care and support of people with disabilities. The coping strategies in this book are as much for caregivers as they are for individuals with disabilities.

What's Stopping You? is also a resource for anyone who works with people with disabilities, including doctors, nurses, physiotherapists, occupational therapists, counsellors, the clergy, and other caregivers. We discuss what to do to obtain the greatest benefit from medical and rehabilitative services, and describe how people with disabilities and their caregivers can work together. We also provide insight into how the identities of people with disabilities can change, and show how these changes can be channelled in positive ways.

What's Stopping You? is also for the individual who wants to plan for his personal and familial well-being. In Chapters 11, 12, and 13, we focus on the strategies you can use to protect yourself legally and financially in the event of a disability. These sections will also be helpful for anyone involved in the process of planning for a disability, such as insurance consultants, financial planners, lawyers, and accountants. Informed professionals can provide families with the advice, care, and coverage they need.

WHAT DO I NEED TO KNOW?

Over the course of this book, we explore a wide range of concerns. Here is a sample of the material we cover, which reflects many of the most frequently asked questions about disability:

- Why did the disability happen?
- Why am I so angry/frustrated?
- How will I cope?
- How will my family respond?
- What will happen to my marriage?
- What obligations do we have to each other?
- Can I still enjoy sex after my disability?
- How can I avoid family break-up?
- What resources are available to help us?
- Where is the best place for me to live?
- What kind of work can I do?
- How can I readjust to the workplace?
- Where do I go for information and counselling?
- How do I select the most appropriate caregivers and treatments?
- How can I work with care providers?
- What are my rights?
- How much will my disability cost?
- Will my insurance cover my expenses?
- What is advocacy and what can it do for me?
- What protection is available and what do I need?
- Where can I go for financial aid?
- How do I plan for my future?
- Can I become independent again?
- Can I help others in similar circumstances?

This book looks at these questions and many more. We have divided the text into three parts. In the first part, we discuss the impact of disability on individuals and families; in the second, we discuss providing care and maximizing care and rehabilitation; and in the third part, we discuss how to build a plan that helps protect you from the consequences of disability.

This is a general disability guide and does not contain detailed information about specific medical conditions. In the appendices, we provide a guide to literature, Web sites, and organizations that can furnish information about a particular medical condition.

CONCLUSION

People with disabilities can do amazing things. They are tremendous fathers, mothers, husbands, wives, partners, and children. People with disabilities are teachers, writers, politicians, executives, athletes, cartoonists, and everything else under the sun. Their accomplishments are constantly defying the traditional belief that people with disabilities are weak, helpless, and dependent. With the love and support of caregivers, a positive attitude, and a good protection plan, anyone can overcome the challenges of disability.

PART 1

Living with

a Disability

Chapter

1

Adjusting to Disability

A POSITIVE ATTITUDE IS ESSENTIAL!

Having the right attitude is the most important part of adjusting to a disability. A disability may force you to re-examine your self-image, your closest relationships, and your role in your family and at work. Making the emotional adjustment to having a disability is often the most difficult task of all, but it is essential to maximizing your quality of life.

A few years ago, I met a businessman named Howard who had the reputation of being extremely efficient and ruthless. He was severely injured in a car accident when a piece of steel penetrated his stomach and rendered his kidneys and his bowels temporarily useless. He woke up after the accident to discover that doctors had performed an ostomy in order to save his life. (An ostomy is a surgery in which the anus is closed on a temporary or permanent basis because it can no longer function properly.) A disposable bag was attached to his abdomen, and he was required to dispose of his personal waste on a regular basis until his anus was reconstructed. When I asked Howard how in the world he contended with the ostomy, he looked right at me and said, "Like in business, when you encounter a barrier, you overcome it. I wanted to get out of the hospital as soon as possible and back into the office. Other than that, I didn't give a f——ing shit."

He makes an obvious but crucial point. You have to commit to doing whatever it takes to surmount your problems. Most people have the potential to assume this attitude, but it is not always easy. Not everyone can be positive, focused, and goal-oriented right off the bat. With disability, so much of your progress depends on your attitude. Take, for example, two people whose legs are crushed in a car accident and who are unable to walk as a result. Each of them faces a painful and difficult road to rehabilitation. The one who is committed to his goal, who goes to every rehab session, and who pushes himself to the absolute maximum may require only a year to walk again. If the other individual despairs at his plight and refuses to commit to rehabilitation, he will make little progress and may never walk again. In this case, the difference lies in their motivation and dedication to rehabilitation.

Why Me?

After being diagnosed with a disability, many people feel sorry for themselves and wonder how they could have been so unlucky. Others question their religious beliefs after being stricken with a serious illness. They feel that they have lived a good life, and have done nothing to deserve these problems. The truth is that disability makes no distinction between people who are good or bad, rich or poor, tall or short. It can strike without warning or explanation.

Disability is not a punishment for something you have done

wrong — it is an event that often has no explanation. It is pointless to dwell on why it happened, because you will never get a satisfactory answer. Turn the question around and ask, "Why not me?"

Why Not Me?

Some people feel that they can deal with any challenge and overcome it. If a very difficult situation emerges, a person with this attitude knows that he has the capacity to deal with anything. Instead of feeling victimized or singled out by fate, he has the confidence to rise to the occasion. Instead of being overwhelmed by the new set of responsibilities, he takes control. He views it as a situation that must be taken care of, and feels that no one could deal with the situation as effectively as he could. Initially, he may not know exactly how to address all of the challenges, but if he has access to the people who can provide him with the information and expertise that he needs, he will be all right. Developing this kind of positive attitude is vital for everyone who encounters disability.

Successful Optimism

An optimist hopes for the best. A successful optimist is someone who not only hopes for the best, but also makes sure that he obtains the best. These are attributes that can help you become a successful optimist, and they capture the mind-set that will best help you cope with a disability:

- A successful optimist will hope and work for the best possible result.
- A successful optimist will always be willing to do more than he is asked.
- A successful optimist believes that he controls his own future.

- A successful optimist focuses on what she can do, rather than on what she can't.
- A successful optimist wants to exceed expectations.
- A successful optimist focuses on the best that can happen, rather than the worst.
- A successful optimist will explore new possibilities and *all* alternatives.
- A successful optimist will seek out and welcome support from all sources.
- A successful optimist will always push himself to exceed his best.
- A successful optimist accepts what cannot be changed.

A positive attitude will ease all facets of coping, and will make any adjustment much easier. If you have confidence and believe in yourself, you will be able to transcend any of the physical or emotional trials you may encounter.

DISABILITY AND SELF-IMAGE

Your self-image can be dramatically affected by a temporary or permanent disability. After a medical crisis occurs, an individual may feel that his identity as a fully functional and contributing member of society has been compromised and violated. In the course of adjusting his self-image to fit with his disability, he may have to reforge his identity to take into account new strengths, weaknesses, and capabilities.

Negotiating a successful change in identity depends on a number of factors. Maturity, experience with highly stressful situations, available social support, age, financial situation, the opportunity to express emotions, and a number of other factors all influence one's ability to adjust to a new identity. These changes can be positive, as illustrated by Stephen Hawking.

Stephen Hawking's Story

Stephen Hawking was on his way to making his mark in the realm of mathematics and theoretical physics when he was diagnosed with Lou Gehrig's disease, a degenerative motor neurone disorder that shuts down your ability to move while leaving your brain and internal organs intact. Since his diagnosis, Professor Hawking has lost the ability to walk, get in and out of bed independently, eat without assistance, and communicate verbally. However, like others who cope with disability effectively, Hawking chooses not to focus on what he cannot do, but rather on what he can do.

Hawking attributes his drive to succeed and to live life to its fullest to the period immediately after his diagnosis. He writes:

My dreams at that time were rather disturbed. Before my condition had been diagnosed, I had been very bored with life. There had not seemed to be anything worth doing. But shortly after I came out of hospital, I dreamt I was going to be executed. I suddenly realised there were a lot of worthwhile things I could do if I were reprieved. Another dream I had several times was that I would sacrifice my life to save others. After all, if I were going to die anyway, it might as well do some good. But I didn't die. In fact, although there was a cloud hanging over my future, I found to my surprise that I was enjoying life in the present more than before. I began to make progress with my research, and I got engaged to a girl called Jane Wilde, who I had met about the time my condition was diagnosed.[1]

---

1 The complete version of Stephen Hawkings's personal story can be found at www.damtp.cam.ac.uk/user/hawking/disability.html.

Professor Hawking approached his disability with optimism rather than depression. Instead of giving up and withdrawing into a shell, he became even more productive. He has published numerous articles and books, including the bestseller *A Brief History of Time*. Since his diagnosis, he has also had three children. He continues to combine his family life and research into theoretical physics with an extensive program of travel and public lectures.

Everyone adjusts to disability in a different way, but some basic steps are typical: getting through the initial recovery and rehabilitation period; making the necessary adjustments in living space, transportation, work, schooling, and financial arrangements; and trying to deal with significant changes in appearance and in family and personal relationships. A person who previously had a well-ordered life may find it turned upside down. He not only has to contend with new limitations, but may also have to cope with the emotional losses caused by sudden and dramatic changes in life goals, future plans, and dreams.

Successful adjustment to disability involves more than mere survival. To successfully survive a major disability, you must go beyond coping with the mental and physical pain, or trying to re-create the sense of normalcy that existed prior to the disability. True survivors are those people who manage to build themselves a new life based on self-awareness and an acknowledgment of personal limitations. To transcend the disability, the survivor must integrate her disability into a new, positive self-image.

There are, however, many obstacles to be overcome on the road to personal recovery. To become whole once again, you must be willing to accept healing as a personal challenge. A serious disability can be an opportunity for positive change. You can find meaning in adversity, but to do so you will have to call upon deep reservoirs of personal strength, and rely on social support from your family and friends.

Resisting Negative Stereotypes

Our body is our most precious possession, and it forms an integral part of our identity. We become familiar with it, learning its capabilities, strengths, and peculiarities. Acceptance of our bodies is taken largely for granted. Physical disability can create a stigma — it marks a person as different and makes them feel as if they exist outside of "normal society." This can have the effect of reducing an individual's self-image from that of a whole, acceptable person to one who is tainted and compromised. Qualities that have no relation to an individual are often attributed to him on the basis of his disability alone. The story of John Merrick, told in *The Elephant Man*, illustrates the way that physical appearances can affect how society treats an individual who is different. In this case, a brilliant, kind man who had severe physical deformities was forced to the margins of society because people were unable to look past his appearance.

Many people who have disabilities are aware, or become aware, of societal attitudes and stereotypes that define people with disabilities as weak, unworthy of responsibility, and incompetent. As a result, they may come to see themselves as damaged and unable to live up to society's expectations. If friends, family, and most important, the individual himself do not guard against this process, the self-image can be devalued. People with a powerful sense of their own abilities and self-worth can protect themselves on their own. With the steadfast support and involvement of family and friends, even people who are initially shaken by their disability can rebound to become confident, secure, and content.

Effective adjustment to disability relies on positive coping mechanisms that enable you to see yourself in a positive light.

Several strategies can aid in this process. You must recognize that the dominant values of society do not have to be the values that are most important to you. You can focus on new values and new physical skills which emphasize your strengths. Learning new skills may enable you to perform the same tasks, in a different fashion, and overcome your limitations.

Although the disability may inconvenience you and limit your range of activities, it does not devalue you as a person. Your entire life does not have to be determined or affected by the disability. **You are not your condition; your condition should be only one part of you.** Don't compare yourself with an absolute, outside scale that is based on what other people seem to be able to do. By shifting your emphasis from specific physical skills onto personality traits that are more relevant to your experience (i.e., resilience, effort, wisdom), you can take pride in having used your capabilities to the maximum.

Successful adjustment may include being able to fend for yourself physically, having control of your emotions, being realistic about your circumstances, continuing to function and carry out personal goals, and maintaining a positive outlook on life. Adjustment to disability is an ongoing process, during which you must develop new skills on a situation-by-situation basis. If you pursue rehabilitation with diligence, you will inspire the support of others and may achieve gains that no one dreamed possible.

Other stresses can also have a dramatic impact on the recovery process. If you have experienced serious crises in your past, you may be more capable of handling a subsequent personal tragedy. One woman, who underwent numerous surgeries as the result of a car accident, wrote, "When I had to go in for an emergency operation because of complications from a previous surgery, I remember facing the prospect of more time confined to a cast, in a wheelchair with an amused, ironic gaiety, the confidence of a survivor." Past experience with illness, disability, and trauma can help you to cope.

The ability to find meaning in your condition is another important ingredient in coping. Ultimately, having a disability is not fun. That does not mean you won't enjoy life, but it is not a challenge that you would choose to undertake. While it's not always easy to work your life around all of the barriers society can erect, it can be done. You do not have to let disability dominate your life or identity.

In the words of a former student:

> *Now that I have distanced myself somewhat from the hospital world, I am able to see more clearly what my own accident has given me. I understand that what I really learned about is suffering. But more importantly, I learned through suffering. My personal odyssey allows me to experience my life with the joy of a Survivor, someone who knows the value of small things. No longer attached to a conception of what I once was, I realize that recovery doesn't mean days of bliss or the end of problems, pain, tears, and hurt. Recovery means learning to accept myself and all parts of myself on an equal basis. I have come to love life with the same intensity I once needed to survive. But the important thing to remember is that there is more to life than simply surviving. It takes a great deal of effort and persistence in spite of ambivalence, fear, and resistance to make it beyond survival.*

Temporary Disability and Self-Image

Even if a disability lasts for only a short period of time, it can still have a significant impact on your life. If you do not have a positive attitude, even minor disabilities can prevent you from getting the most out of life. You must mobilize all of your positive coping skills and family supports to overcome a temporary disability and return to all of your usual activities as soon as possible.

Mary

Mary, the mother of a close friend of mine from Toronto, developed Bell's palsy a week before her daughter's wedding. Bell's palsy is a form of facial paralysis that made it difficult for her to talk, smile, and swallow, and caused nasal drip and uncontrollable drooling. Mary became extremely depressed at the prospect of attending the wedding with a "facial disfigurement." Her family and friends assured her that she would be fine, and that people would understand that she had no control over her condition. Prior to the wedding, she spent an hour and a half with her pastor, who comforted her and convinced her that her disability was irrelevant in the greater scheme of things. She was there to celebrate a joyous occasion with her entire family, and her facial problem was secondary. Mary was very embarrassed during the early part of the reception, but after the dinner and during the party she was able to relax and enjoy the festivities.

After three weeks, her condition and all of its effects disappeared. She no longer felt awkward in social situations, and she resumed all of her former activities. The condition returned twice in the following five years and caused her significant stress each time, but the facial paralysis always disappeared within several weeks. Her positive attitude and the constant support of family and friends were essential to her successful battle with her temporary disability.

Changes to How Others See You

Disability can also bring about significant changes in the way others see you. Strangers and even friends may avoid you, talk down to you, or treat you like a child. To this day, in restaurants, wait staff will sometimes give the bill to my wife or my children, and ask them what I want to eat. These humiliating activities may force a radical attitude readjustment, to prevent others' insensitivity from making you miserable. You have to believe the adage "If they can't accept me for what I am, that's their problem, not mine." I have followed this philosophy for more than fifty years, but to this day it is difficult to adhere to absolutely. On occasion, an insensitive comment or action will still bother me, no matter how hard I try to put it aside. My trip to Paris takes the cake in this respect.

A number of years ago, I was travelling alone across Europe. I planned to spend three days in Paris, seeing the Louvre, the cafés, and many of the beautiful historical landmarks that dot the city. I arrived in the middle of the afternoon and rented a small room on the Left Bank. I was hungry and went for dinner to a charming restaurant in the neighbourhood. I sat down and ordered dinner. I had just finished my appetizer when I was surrounded by two gendarmes, hustled out of the restaurant, and arrested.

I was held overnight in a detention centre filled with a variety of drug dealers, pimps, thieves, and a number of rather large Parisian men, whom I assumed were criminals (although I did not inquire as to their occupation). Until I was brought before a magistrate the next morning, I had no idea why I had been arrested. Apparently, someone at the restaurant had mistaken the tremors caused by my cerebral palsy for the symptoms of heroin withdrawal, and called the police. Fortunately, the magistrate spoke English, and I was able to explain my situation. He made me take my jacket off so he could examine both of my arms for needle marks. Seeing none, he accepted my explanation, ordered my release, and apologized. I returned to my hotel the next morning, and the proprietor said, "You must have had a wonderful night in Paris. Why did you rent the room? You didn't even use it." I shrugged my shoulders and said, "You should only know." With the passage of time, I can look back on this story with a sense of humour, but at the time it was absolutely devastating.

It is unlikely that you will be arrested just for having a disability, but I think my adventure shows the misapprehensions people can have whenever you are "different." Even at home, I have been thrown out of restaurants by owners who thought I was drunk. When I tried to explain my condition, the owners simply refused to listen. I still feel very uncomfortable going into restaurants alone.

Even if you have a positive attitude, adjusting to having a disability may bring on a range of emotions that can create stress and complicate your rehabilitation. These emotions are to be expected, and if you recognize and confront them, you can keep them under control. If you know what to expect, and where the dangers lie, living with a disability can be much easier.

THE RANGE OF EMOTIONS

Shock, paralysis, blame, confusion, depression, and anger are some of the most common reactions felt by people with disabilities. Sometimes these emotions overlap one another, further complicating the process of adaptation. Everyone will experience some or all of these emotions. It is crucial to identify these feelings as soon as they occur, and take the necessary steps to control them. A positive attitude, early recognition, and swift action will enable you to move forward.

Feelings of confusion and depression are a common reaction

to the onset of unforeseen medical problems. If you experience these, remember that you are not alone, and that you have the ability to overcome them.

Shock

Shock is often one of the first emotions people experience. Even if you have been ill for some time, or have a genetic predisposition to a certain condition, a negative diagnosis can still be shocking. The planning and mental preparations you may have made might be insufficient to shield you from the emotional impact of the diagnosis.

Someone who experiences shock may be haunted by horror stories and negative images of disability, leading him to a pessimistic view of the opportunities and potential that exist. You may start to worry about questions that cannot be answered at the time.

Shock can induce temporary paralysis, preventing you from taking action. It can hinder your ability to make rational decisions and difficult choices; in some cases, victims of shock are unable to function. Overcoming shock can take hours, days, weeks, or months, depending on the individual and the extent of their incapacitation. In addition to relying on family and friends for support, you should have people to help with decision-making and your day-to-day responsibilities.

A formal disability plan can help to avert the uncertainty brought on by disability. A financial cushion will give you the time to weigh your options and find the most positive solutions. Designating a power of attorney, as described in the chapter on legal protection, can help clarify decision-making in some scenarios. On a personal level, professional counselling for all family members can be helpful.

Charlene was a twenty-six-year-old mother of three who

worked as an architect. During a routine self-examination, she discovered a lump in her breast. She went to her doctor at once, and he ordered a biopsy. The biopsy revealed that she had breast cancer that may have spread to her bones. She was told that a mastectomy was the only option for survival, and that even then her prognosis was not good. She found this diagnosis shocking. She worried about dying, about how her husband would respond, about how her children would deal with her condition, and about who would take care of them if she died. She also worried about the loss of her femininity and her identity as a woman if her breasts were removed.

She was so overwhelmed by these questions that she did nothing for the first two weeks after the diagnosis. She did not even inform her husband. After this time, the doctor took the initiative, called her husband, and arranged a meeting where they could discuss all the relevant issues. The husband was incredibly supportive, and helped his wife as she underwent surgery, chemotherapy, and radiation treatment. These treatments were successful, and several years later she remains cancer-free. She has re-established her career as an architect, and she also organizes self-help groups for breast cancer survivors.

Extended periods of shock are common, and can delay diagnosis, rehabilitation, and cure. Although this case had a happy ending, the two-week delay between diagnosis and action could have been fatal. It is essential to overcome shock as quickly as possible, both for medical reasons and because prolonged periods of shock can act as a catalyst for other forms of negative coping, such as paralysis.

Paralysis

Discovering that you have what may be a major medical problem can feel like an assault on your entire being. Your health, your self-image, and your self-esteem are all called into question, and the weight of the issues and challenges you have to deal with can be emotionally draining. All of the new information and the flood of emotions you have to process can lead to overload — and create temporary or long-term paralysis. This does not mean that you will be physically unable to move, but you may lose the motivation or the ability to cope with your new challenges.

It is important to begin rehabilitation as soon as possible, as delays in seeking treatment can have a serious, long-term impact. Strokes, cancer, mental illness, hypertension, and a multitude of other conditions must be addressed immediately to achieve the best results. Sometimes, overcoming paralysis is simply a matter of willpower. If you accept the hard road that lies ahead and make the commitment to try to overcome it, you can be successful. However, many patients feel it is too much of a burden and make little effort to help themselves. This is not a recipe for success. If you experience paralysis and do not take concrete steps to overcome your condition, your rehabilitation time will increase, and your physical and mental health may decline.

Sometimes, however, sheer willpower is not enough. You may have to rely on outsiders to help you overcome paralysis. For example, stroke victims are often required to engage in therapy immediately in order to alleviate, and hopefully reverse, their condition. But many stroke victims resign themselves to their situation. The belief that they will not get any better prevents them from engaging in the necessary treatment. Friends and family members must pay close attention to their loved ones, and constantly encourage them to exceed expectations.

Stigma

The stigma associated with some conditions can lead people to avoid treatment. This is often seen in cases of mental illness, as people give in to negative societal attitudes towards conditions such as depression and schizophrenia. Some people refuse to acknowledge their problem or seek treatment out of fear that people may find out and label them "crazy." If this response is allowed to continue, the symptoms can intensify and become harder to treat. Care facilities recognize these difficulties and are taking steps to make it easier to gain access to treatment. The key step is to overcome a patient's initial unwillingness or inability to enter a care program, and let the healing begin. No one should feel that they are less of a person because they have a mental illness.

Max was a nineteen-year-old who worked three jobs to pay his way through university. He was a short-order cook at two different McDonald's and a Burger King. In his first two years at university, he was able to keep up this hectic pace, earning a B average on a full course load. In his third year, however, he began to engage in increasingly bizarre behaviour, and eventually stripped himself naked on the public transportation system and was taken into custody. He underwent a thorough examination and was diagnosed with schizophrenia. He was hospitalized for two months and received outpatient treatment for the following three months. After these five months, he was told that he could control his condition through drug therapy and ongoing therapeutic counselling. His doctors also suggested reducing his course load and his excessive work hours.

Max was uncomfortable returning to school in his home town. He felt that everyone looked at him differently, and just thought of him as "that guy who stripped on the subway." As a result, he left his family and friends and moved 2,000 miles away, to go to school in another community where no one was aware of his mental illness and no one would place labels on him. After several months in his new community, where he had no contact with mental-health support services, nor with friends and family, he suffered a complete nervous breakdown and was hospitalized for a second time. The stigma that was attached to mental illness had caused him to remove himself from a protective and supportive environment, and place himself into one in which he was more vulnerable to his condition.

Stigma can also lead to delays in treatment. Patients with HIV, AIDS, cancer, or mental illnesses sometimes feel ashamed or embarrassed and are reluctant to seek care. Even short delays can exacerbate your condition. Rejecting the stereotypes attached to certain conditions is an essential step in coping. Friends, family members, and medical personnel can minimize the impact of stigma, and encourage their loved ones to engage in therapy as long as it is necessary.

Blame

Whenever a disability occurs, there is a tendency to try to find someone to blame. This is a common human reaction, but it is rarely productive. A disability often has no identifiable cause, so days, weeks, and months can be lost in the fruitless pursuit of a scapegoat. Focus your energy on improving your health, not on finding someone to punish.

If your disability is a result of negligence or a blatant disregard for your well-being, however, it may be worthwhile to pursue legal action. A successful lawsuit, settlement, or criminal prosecution can have several effects: it can provide closure or satisfaction that the person responsible was brought to justice; it can protect others from being victimized; and it can provide financial benefits. If you do pursue legal action, however, try to ensure that it does not become all-consuming, and overwhelm your greater goal of enjoying a high quality of life.

Henry was a dockworker from Detroit. He was injured by a front-end loader at work and sued his company for negligence. The impact of his injuries was largely invisible (back pain, leg pain, dizziness, memory loss), which made it very difficult to confirm his diagnosis. He spent countless hours on the telephone and in meetings with his attorneys and insurance advisers, and dedicated very little time to his prescribed rehabilitation program. He focused almost all of his efforts on "making the company pay" for his injuries, wasted thousands of dollars on legal fees, and fixated on his crusade to the point that he developed depression. After several years, he received a small settlement of $40,000, more than half of which was consumed by legal expenses.

If Henry had concentrated on rehabilitation and retraining instead of his lawsuit, he could have avoided large amounts of stress and his bouts of depression. He may even have been able to return to his own job much earlier. Focus on tasks that will enhance your rehabilitation and reintegration — don't get bogged down in the hunt for recrimination.

Confusion

The pressures of making unfamiliar choices can lead to indecisiveness and uncertainty. Disability can lead to increased job, family, and financial stress, and raise a number of questions that you never thought of before. When facing these unfamiliar situations, people often make hasty decisions before investigating the consequences. Because confusion can lead to poor decision-making, it is important to understand what you require, and to take a logical approach to meeting your needs. Imposing a structure on your problems allows you to deal with them in order of priority and with a clear mind; if you are aware of the pros and cons, you can minimize confusion. If you plan in advance and have a safety net to fall back on, you will have the time to refocus your priorities and goals, and make adjustments.

Over the course of their care, patients are often given a wide variety of options. It is not unusual for patients who are diagnosed with fibromyalgia to have to choose between four or five different medical programs, for example. If you have just learned of your condition and are not a medical expert, selecting from a wide range of treatment strategies can be daunting and confusing. Unless you are facing an emergency, you should step back and consider each option carefully. Taking your time will give you confidence in your decision.

Sometimes, however, a patient discovers that what worked for one group of patients does not work for him. This can lead to frustration and disappointment, and can cause a patient to wonder if he or his physician has done something wrong. By taking responsibility for your treatment, and carefully tracking and noting your reaction to your medications and therapies, you can help your physician to develop a new course of care. Instead of being mystified as to what went wrong, you and your physician can clearly assess your reactions and move forward with confidence.

Depression

If you are facing surgery, many hours of intense rehabilitation and treatment, or the possibility that you may not be able to work for an extended period of time, you may be at risk of depression. These thoughts can be compounded by feelings of isolation and stigmatization. A strong family and support structure can combat these emotions, but sometimes professional help is required. Counselling is an excellent strategy for people who feel depressed. Open discussions of your feelings with a qualified and empathetic professional can help you to emerge from these difficult periods. Antidepressant medication is also appropriate in some cases.

Darren worked as a cab driver to put himself through law school. He graduated as an A student and was engaged to be married. He articled for a year and was looking forward to establishing his own practice. He had experienced arthritis-like symptoms for the preceding five years, however, and as he was about to start out on his own, he began to experience pain throughout his body. He went to a medical clinic for a full examination and was diagnosed with scleroderma, a connective tissue disease for which there is no known cure. He had never heard of scleroderma before, and he had no idea of the implications of his diagnosis. For the next two weeks, he was extremely depressed. He read whatever he could find on scleroderma and went to see numerous doctors for second opinions. His depression deepened when he realized that the condition was terminal, and he considered giving up his career in law.

Darren relied heavily on his family during this time. They were unbelievably supportive, and reminded him that he had excelled in law school and should not give up on his dreams. His fiancée told him that he could overcome anything, and that she would stand by him. After a month of reflection, he realized that he was not going to let the disability stand in his way. He emerged from his depression rededicated to the practice of law and to his fiancée, whom he subsequently married. He went on to establish a thriving practice and develop a sterling reputation, and was cited by a trial judge for his "diligence, insight, and compassion." Darren worked as a lawyer for fifteen years before he had to retire because of the scleroderma. He refused to give in to the disappointment of a terminal diagnosis, and he lived life to its fullest.

Anger

Venting your emotions to a caregiver or confidant is important. It always helps to have someone with whom you can share all of your emotions — joy, anger, sadness — anything. A confidant can prevent anger and rage from accumulating, and can avert nasty outbursts and tantrums that could permanently damage relationships. If you do not have an outlet for your frustrations, you may unknowingly lash out at friends, family members, and even caregivers. Focus your anger on overcoming the problems you face, and use it as a motivational tool to attain greater achievements.

Anger can also be a barrier to treatment. People become angry at the doctors who have diagnosed them, but instead of lashing out at the doctors, they reject the treatment they have been offered — to their own detriment. Sometimes the intervention of family and friends only increases the anger, and hardens the patient's resolve not to engage in treatment. For example, I knew a patient who became depressed and angry following a stroke. He refused to undertake any rehabilitation, and as a result he spent the rest of his life living with the maximum impact of the stroke. What could have been a treatable medical set-back became an insurmountable barrier. If he had set aside his anger and embraced an intensive therapeutic program, he could have overcome almost all of the effects of the stroke. If you are angry about your disability, do not lash out or reject the help that you are offered. Channel all of your energy into rehabilitation, into fighting the disease or disability with all of your heart and soul. Instead of screaming at someone, exercise until you don't have the energy to yell. Rage can be a powerful weapon if used properly.

Self-Isolation

Sometimes people who suffer disabilities feel ashamed and angry, and try to cut themselves off from the world. They push away loved ones and antagonize anyone who tries to help. Some people become hermits because of their illness, rejecting their family and friends because they are unhappy with themselves. Many individuals give in psychologically long before they give in physically.

Denise was a homemaker and mother of two who had been married for more than twenty years. She was an active volunteer for the United Way and the Heart and Stroke Foundation. When she reached her early forties, she began to experience painful and debilitating headaches. When the headaches struck, they caused her to lose her sight, and on occasion she would experience partial paralysis. She went to her physician, who ordered a wide range of tests. She was diagnosed with brain cancer, and three different physicians confirmed her terminal condition. Her diagnosis made her very angry and depressed, and she chose to cut herself off from her family and friends. Her rage led her to hurt her loved ones by isolating herself.

Resist the desire to push away your family and friends during your time of need. They will be the rock that you can cling to. In fact, these times can be opportunities for you to strengthen your relationships with the people around you. People whom you may have never relied on or felt close to may surprise you with the depth of their understanding and support. Phenomenal people are there to reach out to you, but they must be given the opportunity.

Some people are able to take a positive approach to any situation, even a terminal condition. My late mother-in-law had breast cancer that metastasized into bone cancer, a condition that was very painful. She also developed lung cancer. In the final year of her life, she always had a smile on her face in spite of incredible pain, and she seldom, if ever, talked about her impending death. On the last day of her life she had a party in her hospital room, during which she said a warm goodbye to her family and her close friends. She was even stronger than all of us.

In these dramatic situations you have a choice. You can feel sorry for yourself, or you can deal with the information as my mother-in-law did — by accepting the inevitable and rising above it. She set an example with her courage, and inspired her friends and family to carry on. By refusing to give in to self-pity, she eased the grieving process for her loved ones.

A very good friend of mine, who passed away before he was thirty-five, told his wife that it was unacceptable for her to mourn for him for the rest of her life. He said that for the sake of her life and that of their children, she must resume a "normal" life after a suitable period of reflection and mourning. This involved marrying again. As a matter of fact, my friend told his wife that if she didn't remarry, he would come back to haunt her. She took his advice, and a few years after the death of her first husband, she married a wonderful man.

It is important to share your zest for life with your loved ones. Many people with terminal conditions take family vacations in their last few months of life in order to enjoy their time to the fullest, and to leave their loved ones with positive memories. Sharing your courage and spirit by persevering in the face of a tremendous challenge serves as an inspiration. You want family members to be prepared to move on after a period of mourning, rather than have their lives come to a standstill after the death. Letting family and caregivers know how important their efforts have been can go a long way to easing the mourning process.

EXPRESSING YOUR EMOTIONS

Earlier in this chapter, we mentioned the need for you to have someone with whom you can share your innermost emotions, and this point needs to be emphasized. Sometimes you simply have to express your emotions. If you channel it into the right outlet, even anger can be a positive emotion. For example, I know a woman who experienced a tremendous sense of rage and anger after she was diagnosed with breast cancer. After she received the diagnosis, she went home and entered her garage. Over the next ten minutes, she took 150 clay pots and smashed them against a cement wall.

This physical expression of her emotions enabled her to move past her anger. The next day, she went to her oncologist and began treatment. Not everyone will express their emotions the same way (few people own that many pots), but expressing yourself through physical action can be therapeutic. Make sure, however, that you do not endanger yourself or anyone else when expressing your emotions. Don't make other people the focal point of your anger, and don't vent these emotions in a potentially dangerous situation (i.e., while driving or handling a firearm). Professional therapists are also appropriate people with whom you can vent your emotions.

BARRIERS TO ADJUSTMENT

There are a number of other problems that people with disabilities may confront. If you are aware of these obstacles, it is easier to surmount them.

Expectations

Make sure that you select the appropriate goal or series of goals. You don't want to set your limits too low; too many people limit what they attempt to achieve because experts tell them more can't be done. The people who have made the most monumental gains after a disability are those who refused to allow the expectations of others to define what they could accomplish.

Stan was an active golfer, swimmer, and tennis player. He belonged to a private club in Vancouver and played sports year-round. He lost control of his car on black ice while driving home one day, and hit a telephone pole. He was freed from the wreck, but his arm had to be amputated. Stan was told that in all likelihood, he would not be able to play any of the sports he loved because of his artificial arm. He was stunned by this diagnosis, as these games had been an important part of his life since childhood. After a few months, he decided that he knew better than his doctors. He disregarded the diagnosis and began a very determined plan of rehabilitation, focusing on learning how to play all of his favourite sports with his prosthetic arm. After a year-long period of rehabilitation, he was able to swim well, play tennis, and break one hundred on the golf course. His determination enabled him to far surpass his physician's expectations.

Some professionals and family members become convinced that the impact of a disability will be significant and total. The belief that there is little hope for improvement can become a self-fulfilling prophecy: people who believe that they cannot make their life better are unwilling to take the steps that *will* make their life better. The opposite is also true. Belief in yourself will be reinforced many times over. Be optimistic while remaining realistic about your opportunities for progress and integration. Maintain faith in yourself, even if other people have doubts.

Realistic Expectations

Always try to surpass the barrier that is set as your upper limit of achievement, but at the same time be realistic about your choices. For example, if you are a social worker who becomes a paraplegic at forty years of age, you can probably make several adjustments and continue with your career. If you had a similar injury but were in a profession that required significant manual dexterity, it is unlikely that you would be able to continue your career. When it is appropriate, you should refocus your efforts toward other areas.

In my case, I was told early on in life that owing to my cerebral palsy, I would never have the physical ability to write. Instead of spending hundreds of hours and thousands of dollars on treatments with little chance of success, I focused on maximizing my strengths and working on other physical skills. My disability has not prevented me from becoming a university professor or from publishing eight books. There are some things I may have to concede to my disability (I would never have made it as a professional athlete, for example), but in the academic field I have surpassed the expectations of many of the teachers and professors who told me that I would never be a success.

If you have just experienced disability, you may have to re-evaluate your strengths. Learning about your condition will allow you to determine what opportunities exist and what strategies will enable you to make the most significant gains. Push your limits without getting sidetracked in hopeless endeavours. I have climbed mountains, but I will never be able to thread a needle. So I pay a tailor to do my sewing, and I enjoy the view from up high.

Playing the Percentages

People always ask doctors and therapists what their chances are. They feel that being given a number will provide insight into their chances of getting better. Unfortunately, many numbers are meaningless. For example, when a doctor tells an accident victim that he has a 50 percent chance of walking again, several problems can emerge. First of all, the prediction may not be accurate. A doctor's estimate may fail to take into account a patient's strength, dedication, or level of support. If an individual is not committed to a rehabilitation program, he may have less than a 10 percent chance of walking again. But if he always does more than is required by his therapist, his chances may improve to more than 90 percent. Many professionals do not like giving numbers because the percentage they cite may be only an average or an educated guess, which doesn't take into account key individual factors.

Percentages can also discourage people from realizing their potential. If a doctor or therapist gives you a very low chance of reaching a certain goal, it can be discouraging and can eliminate the desire to rehabilitate. Sometimes a patient will say, "If only one person in twenty in my condition can do it, why bother?" Instead of asking for a percentage, you should ask, "What is the best that I can hope for?" This way, you will be alerted to the possibilities of success and not set up for failure.

The Danger of Labelling

Labels can cause many problems, including stereotyping. Resisting labels is essential to avoiding prejudice. Predetermined definitions should not prevent you from getting the care, treatment, and acceptance that you deserve.

The mass media have traditionally conveyed negative images of disability, which have led to labelling. For example, the quadriplegic community across America was outraged by the movie *Whose Life Is It Anyway?* This film depicted a man who experienced quadriplegia as the result of an automobile accident, and whose quest in the movie was to take his own life. The movie implied that anyone with quadriplegia who had control over his life would choose to end it, since he had nothing to contribute to society and nothing to live for.

This image is false. Many people with quadriplegia lead active, fulfilling, and independent lives, but the movie established an image that has been tough to dispel. *Whose Life Is It Anyway?* made life more difficult for people who were living with quadriplegia, as they had to deal with the mistaken assumptions of people who believed that the lives of quadriplegics had little meaning. But as long as you have a positive outlook on life and a strong self-image, you will be able to transcend encounters with people whose views of disability belong in the past.

Misconceptions

In some cases, the problems encountered by a person with a disability are imposed not by his physical condition, but by the incorrect assumptions of others. Prejudice, discrimination, social ostracism, and inappropriate comments are all frequent problems faced by people with disabilities. You might think that children are the only ones who make offensive comments, but they are not. People of all ages can be insensitive.

A thick skin helps a lot. When most people make hurtful comments, they are not being malicious, but are usually ignorant or naive. Sometimes, it is best to ignore these comments, or to walk out of a room if you have had enough. If you feel strongly about a particular comment, challenge the person who made it to justify his remarks. People have no right to treat anyone poorly because of a disability. It is most effective to respond to blatant mistreatment in a factual, dispassionate way. Wit can also be an effective tool.

A woman in a wheelchair was showing pictures of her three children at a convention. Someone asked her how she had them, and she wanted to respond, "By f——ing, how else!" But she did not. Instead, she told him, "There are three ways of conceiving.

The first, and hopefully best, way is by making love with your partner. The second is in-vitro fertilization. The third way to conceive a child is through immaculate conception. When I became pregnant, it was immaculate." Not everyone will choose this approach to dealing with people who make ignorant comments, but it can certainly make a lasting impression.

CONCLUSION

Moving into an active, problem-solving mind-set as soon as a condition is diagnosed is the best strategy you can adopt to enhance your quality of life. All of your emotions are natural reactions to a stressful situation, and nothing that you feel during this time is the "wrong" emotion. Everyone requires a period of adjustment, and with time, commitment, support, and love, the negative emotions you feel can be replaced by positive ones. Your family will be an essential part of this process.

Chapter 2

Changing Relationships: Disability, Family, and Friends

INTRODUCTION

I never could have succeeded without the love and support of my family. They always encouraged me to go for it. My dad used to say that most things are possible, some things are extremely difficult, and if something really appears impossible, there may be other ways to achieve the same result. Because of my cerebral palsy, my sense of balance was very poor. Today I still have difficulty performing fine motor tasks. I did not learn to walk until I was five, and have never learned to write. My parents said, "It's a waste of time to put any effort into learning how to write. You can have people write for you. Concentrate on the tasks that you can do or will be able to do, and that are important."

One of the things that many people told my parents would be impossible was for me to learn how to ride a bike. Starting when I was six, my father and his friends worked with me intensively for three years, and by the time I was nine, I learned how to ride.

This was just one of the "impossible" tasks that my family helped me accomplish.

My family was just as essential following my two heart attacks and my double-bypass surgery. My wife, Sharon, and my son David were with me in the hospital every day for many hours. They gave me the courage to face life-threatening surgery, and walked with me in the hospital many times after my surgery, encouraging me to build my endurance. When I returned home, I was still very weak, and Sharon and David helped me with many of the things I would normally do on my own, such as gardening, barbecuing, shopping, and running errands. Sharon joined a cardiac exercise group with me, and she motivated me to participate in this program, which ran for one hour a day, three days a week. Their dedication gave me the confidence to stick to my rigorous rehabilitation schedule, and I became strong enough to resume my teaching career the following September.

Their efforts on my behalf were exceptional, but they were not atypical or unique. Thousands of people achieve their rehabilitative potential with the encouragement of their friends, family, and fellow workers. Family members who provide such vital care aren't heroes — they are average people going about the daily business of living who can call on vast reservoirs of strength to help pull you through. You may never appreciate the strength of your family until it is tested by an unforeseen medical problem.

A disability involves the entire family. It can change how you see one another, the roles you play, and your responsibilities. A disability can change a family's standard of living, and force each member to make sacrifices. With the proper preparation and management, you can handle any pressures that may develop. This chapter describes the changes that can arise with disability and illustrates how a family can successfully adapt.

WHY ARE FAMILIES SO IMPORTANT?

You need people around you whom you can trust and who can help you feel loved, secure, and protected. Your family and closest friends are the ones who will support you throughout your disability, and who will provide you with strength that you probably didn't know you had.

In addition to providing support and encouragement, families fulfil a wide variety of roles. They can provide you with important advice and may be called on to make vital decisions if you are unable to do so. A family member's responsibilities may include:

- authorizing medical treatment and surgery;
- making decisions concerning resuscitation and life support;
- arranging organ transplants and organ donations;
- helping to choose rehabilitation and therapy programs;
- helping to choose short- and long-term care facilities or other living environments;
- providing financial support, making financial transactions, and taking financial responsibility for the household;
- hiring personal-care assistants.

Involve your family whenever possible in decision-making and planning for a disability. Members of your family must be made aware of your wishes so they can respond to your needs accordingly. By installing an appropriate disability protection plan, you can help your family members concentrate on your care without having to worry about the financial implications of your disability.

My family provided the most supportive environment I could have imagined, and they are by no means unique. Here is the

story of another family whose love and support were funda-
mental to their daughter's success in overcoming disability.

Peggy

Peggy was a high-school student whom I had the pleasure of
working with in a support group for people with disabilities.
She was an avid athlete, playing basketball and running track
for her high school. She was also an active volunteer with a
group that donated their hair to have wigs made for young girls
who lost theirs as the result of cancer-related therapy. It was her
ambition to become a police officer who specialized in settling
family disputes, just like her father. At the age of fifteen, though,
Peggy became a paraplegic as the result of a shooting accident.
Her family provided her with constant love and support, and
transported her to and from high school every day. Her brother,
sister, and parents helped her with shopping, bathing, and many
of the other tasks she had to learn anew. They encouraged her
to pursue post-secondary education, and did everything to promote her independence and integration. They encouraged her
to continue her extra-curricular activities, and she took up
wheelchair basketball and horseback riding. She was very successful in both pursuits. Peggy relinquished her dream of
becoming a police officer, but went to university, where she lived
in residence and earned a bachelor of commerce degree with
a B+ average. On graduation, her parents gave her a van that
was retrofitted so she could drive herself to work, shop, and
do everything that she needed on her own. Peggy worked for
three years as a bank teller before she was promoted to the position of loans manager, and she is now happily married. She faces
a number of barriers as the result of her disability, particularly
in terms of recreation, but she refuses to let disability disrupt
her life. Peggy's family provided the support that gave her the

time to adjust to her disability and to learn how to live independently.

THE EXTENDED FAMILY

Look beyond your immediate family for support. Our concept of "family," the people whom you can count on any time of the day or night, is better understood as a "circle of friends." Your circle of friends can include your partner, parents, siblings, other relatives, friends, and acquaintances. We all need people that we can count on, and the more people who can play this role for you, the better.

This example illustrates how a circle of friends can provide support. A group of five married couples met each other for the first time living in a seniors' complex. They shared many activities and interests, and became close friends. They ranged in age from the late sixties to the late seventies. One of the members of the group had already had a heart attack, and another had severe back and hip problems. They realized that because of their ages, some or all of them were likely to experience serious medical difficulties and disabilities within the next several years. They began to contemplate all of the possible scenarios that could occur if one or more of them were to become incapacitated. Each of these couples had raised children who were now adults and were spread all over North America. They realized that none of their children lived close enough to be able to act as a caregiver.

This group of couples designed a "mutual benefit support system" in which they defined a wide range of responsibilities that they would carry out for one another. They started doing all of their shopping together, and they even bought four new cars at the same time — earning a substantial discount. They shared financial strategies and advice, and hired the same housekeeper to clean and maintain all of their apartments.

Tom, a member of the group who had been an architect and a political activist, began to exhibit the early stages of Alzheimer's, forgetting names, occasionally getting lost when he went out for walks, and not remembering to perform basic personal grooming tasks. However, because of the intensive involvement of the group, who always reminded him and encouraged him to do the things he had to do, many of the severe difficulties associated with Alzheimer's have not yet appeared. To this day, the group maintains a high level of activity, enjoying meals and vacations together, playing cards, attending concerts, plays, and movies, swimming, and walking.

Not every support system will be as organized as the one we illustrated. But if your family and friends are committed, caring, and reliable, you will be okay.

TELLING YOUR FAMILY ABOUT A DISABILITY

Telling your loved ones about an illness or disability can be difficult. A straightforward approach may be tough over the short term, but your honesty will pay long-run dividends. Here are several guidelines you can follow to make it easier to share the news of your disability with your family.

- **Try to stay calm and confident.** Your family will respond to your emotions. If you show them you are in control, they will be reassured.
- **Be as open and as honest as possible.** The truth may shock or hurt in the short term, but sharing with your family can minimize uncertainty and help you move on to more important matters.
- **Share accurate information.** You may want to have your physician help you explain the medical aspects of your condition. Providing your family with a clear understanding

of your condition will protect them from uncertainty and anxiety.

- **Have a plan.** Don't just drop a bombshell on your family. Telling them you have a disability can frighten them if it is not accompanied by a strategy that you plan to follow to combat your illness or injury. If you can, say, "I have a disability, but I am doing A, B, and C to help me get better." Demonstrating that you have a plan will give your family confidence, and will encourage their co-operation and participation. You may not have a detailed plan right away, but letting your family know that you are working with medical professionals to create an effective blueprint can have the same effect.

- **Let family members know you need them.** Many people are shy. You will have friends and family members who want to help but who will be reluctant to initiate support. They may not feel comfortable with disability, or may not want to "intrude." Let your family members know that their contributions are valued, and that you want them to be involved.

- **Keep them posted.** Keep your family abreast of your progress once you have told them about your disability. Open lines of communication help keep people involved. Your efforts will encourage the people interested in your care. This will help caregivers feel more connected and enthusiastic, and then they are more likely to be ready when called upon.

Young Children and Disability

Younger children may not even notice or comprehend your new limitations. If this is the case you may not have to tell them. As they grow older, they will just need a simple explanation about your condition. If you experience an instantaneous disability, however, a prompt explanation is essential in order to maintain trust with your kids. If you come home one day in a wheelchair, your children will notice. Even if your disability is "invisible" (i.e., epilepsy), most children will be able to pick up on the fact that something is wrong. You don't have to get into the medical specifics. Emphasize the positives — that you still love them and can care for them, and that although you will have to make some changes, your family will be as strong and successful as before.

A more detailed description of your condition may be warranted when your kids get older. Always speak to them in an open and direct manner — kids know when something is wrong. If they know what you are going through, they will admire and support you.

Walter

Walter worked as an electrical engineer. When he was forty-seven, he was diagnosed with Lou Gehrig's disease (ALS). At the time, his son was five and his daughter fourteen. Walter's doctor informed him that although an exact prognosis was not possible, he probably had at least ten years to live. Initially, he told his youngest child very little, except that "Dad was ill" and required a lot of rest. Walter and his wife, Susan, shared the details of his condition with their daughter, as they believed she was old enough to understand. A full explanation of the disease helped her to accept her father's condition and enabled her to contribute to his care. Over the years, the parents told the son what they believed to be appropriate, and by the time he was ten the boy was fully aware of his father's terminal condition. Being honest and forthright helped keep the family together and strengthened their ability to cope.

TALKING ABOUT DISABILITY WITH FRIENDS AND EXTENDED FAMILY

You are not obligated to do so, but talking about your disability with your friends and extended family can be helpful. Telling them yourself will prevent them from developing misconceptions about your condition and from relying on rumours or gossip. Sharing information can help your friends to understand what you are going through. If they are not aware of your condition, they cannot offer their assistance. You might be overwhelmed by the heartfelt support you receive from your closest friends, and perhaps even from individuals whom you may have considered to be casual acquaintances.

What If I Don't Want to Tell People?

You may feel that your disability is your business and no one else's. It is a perfectly legitimate reaction, and you have every right to protect your privacy. If an acquaintance or a stranger asks, "Is anything wrong?" or "I heard you were ill. Is this true?" a simple response is to dismiss your condition as unimportant, and to move on to another topic of conversation. If people continue to badger you for information, tell them your personal health is a private matter that you would prefer not to discuss, and change the subject.

THE IMPACT OF DISABILITY ON THE FAMILY

Disability can be a huge turning-point for any family. The families that cope the best take an organized approach. Designing an effective plan of care and clearly delineating responsibilities can minimize disruptions to your family's routine. A haphazard approach can put the quality of your care at risk. This story is an example of how a family's planning helped.

Hazel worked as a secretary for a number of years, and then

became a housewife who raised three wonderful children. Her mother and three of her brothers had experienced profound hearing loss at ages ranging from forty to sixty-five. Because doctors had said that her family's problems were probably hereditary, Hazel realized that she was at a very high risk of losing her hearing. She discussed the implications with her family, and they talked about the innovations her siblings had made and about how their home could be adapted if she experienced similar problems. At sixty-one, she began to have a great deal of difficulty talking on the phone and following conversations when she was in a crowd of people. She went to her audiologist at once to design a treatment plan.

Her family installed a specially designed phone that would flash brightly when it rang. They also installed a system of lights that would let Hazel know when the doorbell rang or when the smoke detector had been activated. She bought headphones that enabled her to continue to enjoy radio, television, and classical music. She learned to lip read. Whenever she went out, Hazel brought along a friend — she was worried that she would not be able to hear traffic, and would put herself at risk. For the same reason, she voluntarily gave up her licence.

Although by the age of seventy she had only minimal hearing ability, she maintained a high level of activity with her friends and family, and continued to bowl, hike, and swim. Hazel's discussions with her family were essential to her smooth transition. Her family accepted the disability with ease, and they were able to talk about problems that might arise well in advance and sketch out plans to adapt to her hearing loss. Hazel recognized the importance of these discussions. She told me, "Like the boy scouts, I was prepared."

Hazel's family were ready and willing to make adjustments to accommodate her needs. Not every family makes such an easy transition to disability. Jacob was an insurance adjuster in his mid-forties who developed multiple sclerosis. He and his family were very active and enjoyed numerous outdoor activities, such as hiking, camping, and golf. Jacob was forced to curtail most of these activities when the MS decreased his physical stamina and ability to exercise. His wife, Cherie, refused to make any changes in her lifestyle, however, and continued all of her outdoor activities with the children. As a result, he felt abandoned. Jacob's condition worsened and he became very angry at his wife's failure to be sympathetic. She said, "Just because Dad can no longer do these activities doesn't mean that we have to sit at home and mope." She failed to adjust to the situation by modifying her activities to include her husband more frequently. Jacob's frustration got to the point where he insisted that he and his wife go into counselling to bridge the gap in their relationship.

If disability prevents you from continuing certain activities you used to participate in as a family, you have several alternatives. You don't necessarily have to give up the activities you can no longer do together. But everyone will have to make some concessions to their own desires and schedules. If you carry on as if nothing has happened, or if you refuse to make allowances for the disability, tensions in your family can be exacerbated. Scaling back the activities that exclude one family member and looking for new activities that you can all do together will help you cope.

Although it is difficult to gauge, the partner without a disability should push his spouse to try to continue with as many physical and social activities as possible. Many people with disabilities withdraw from their favourite pursuits before it is necessary, and this can lead to physical or emotional decline. Family members who exhibit negative reactions to disability are often coping with the stress and shock of your diagnosis.

Frequently, such reactions will dissipate as family members come to have a greater understanding of the disability. If these reactions do not change over time, counselling may be appropriate.

There are a number of positive strategies, in addition to counselling, that you can employ to help your family cope.

POSITIVE FAMILY COPING STRATEGIES

Advance Planning

Discussing the possible consequences of a disability when you are healthy can make it easier to adjust to a medical crisis. There are several issues to be addressed:

1. your level of financial protection and your financial capacity to survive disability;
2. what you can expect from each other in terms of care;
3. what you would do in a worst-case scenario (i.e., organ donation, life support, care in the event of a severe disability).

These are serious issues, and they are an essential part of a lifetime commitment. If you avoid these questions, you are doing a great disservice to both yourself and your partner. These questions are discussed in detail in Part 2: Caring for People with Disabilities, and Part 3: Protecting Your Future.

Discuss All Aspects of Your Care

After a disability has occurred, it is essential to discuss the alternatives with your partner and with other family members. You should discuss both short-term issues, such as the selection of caregivers and medical facilities, and long-term issues, such as rehabilitation plans, new career goals, and adapting to new roles within the family. These issues are discussed in more detail later in this book.

Spirituality

Religious belief has helped countless people overcome their disabilities. Belief in a higher power can help patients and caregivers go on in the face of great challenges. Don't underestimate the importance of self-contemplation, religious counselling, meditation, and the support offered within religious communities. Congregations of all faiths offer special programs for those living with illness and disability. Religious groups also provide the opportunity to meet people who are going through similar experiences, and to reach out for their support.

Love and Sexuality

Love and sexuality are an important part of any healthy relationship, and people with disabilities have the same desires and needs as anyone else. Many individuals with serious disabilities continue to enjoy the pleasures of intimacy, which helps them maintain their self-image and their connection to their partner and to society. Disability is no reason to cease physical intimacy.

Even the most serious disabilities may not be a barrier to the enjoyment of physical pleasure. Many people with paraplegia, quadriplegia, and muscular sclerosis, for example, are engaged in fulfilling sexual relationships. Sometimes sexual activity can take alternative and creative forms, emphasizing touching, physical closeness, and massage. Some people are reluctant to re-establish physical bonds until they are comfortable with their new self-image. A partner should remain patient and accept that it may take time. For example, a woman who underwent a double mastectomy was completely unwilling to consider sexual contact with her husband following the surgery. She even felt insecure about his seeing her naked. However, after a month had passed, she was able to overcome her initial trepidation, and they gradually resumed sexual activity. She has told me that their sexual intimacy has become far more meaningful than it was before. It confirmed both her femininity and the depth of her relationship with her husband.

NEGATIVE COPING WITHIN THE FAMILY

Sometimes the stresses of coping and caregiving can lead to negative adaptations. If these behaviours are identified quickly, they are far easier to address. If you are aware of the warning signs, you will be able to put a halt to these behaviours as quickly as possible.

Pity and Overindulgence

Many friends and family members do not know how to respond when a loved one encounters a serious disability. They may yield to stereotypical notions that people with disabilities are dependent and need to be indulged. Most people who have disabilities do not want to be pitied or coddled. If your family and caregivers begin to be indulgent and overprotective, let them know right away. Even though you may require a great deal of support and assistance, let them know that you want to be as independent as possible. People who try to do everything for you mean well and believe that they are helping you, but by taking away your independence and your opportunities to try new activities, they are hindering your rehabilitation.

Nadine was an avid mountain climber. She was on a climbing vacation in the Rocky Mountains, and fell during a tough climb. Nadine lost the use of her right arm and leg, and also injured her left arm. She required several months of intensive physiotherapy before she could even lift a glass with her left arm. Nadine worked hard at her rehabilitation program, lifting light weights and spending hours squeezing a ball with her usable hand, in the attempt to regain muscle strength. Nadine was a very independent person who resented having things done for her. It was a tough adjustment; her friends and family members were required to help her perform the most basic of tasks in the weeks immediately following her accident. During her first two months at home, she was unable to take herself to the washroom or feed herself, but she made rapid progress. However, even after Nadine was able to perform many of these tasks herself, her family and friends continued to perform them for her, as they could do the tasks more quickly and wanted to be helpful.

Nadine was distressed by this unwanted assistance, and she felt dehumanized by her caregivers' actions. Whenever they performed a task that she could do herself, she felt useless. She wanted to take advantage of every opportunity to be independent, but she could not. In the end, she slowly gained the confidence to tell her friends and family when their assistance was not needed. After four years of dedicated rehabilitation, she became totally self-reliant.

Caregivers may find it hard to resist the desire to help their loved ones. But while people with disabilities may not be able to perform some tasks and may often require help, it is essential that they be pushed to their limits and not use their caregivers' assistance as a crutch. Some people with disabilities are tempted to take the easy way out and let aides perform tasks they could do on their own. Discourage this sort of behaviour, and constantly focus on encouraging independence.

Taking Away Independence

After a disability occurs, family members sometimes believe it is their responsibility to assume total control over all facets of your existence. Some caregivers may believe that you have lost the capacity to make decisions about your own care. Their actions are usually well meaning, and are enhanced by the fact that they love you deeply. In fact, many caregivers wonder how trying to make someone's life easier could be a bad thing. This misunderstanding is very common.

If you feel that your caregivers have taken away your independence, express your dissatisfaction directly but with tact and restraint. Make it clear that it is your life, and that you are capable of making significant decisions. Even though it can be frustrating, try to avoid emotional outbursts. Your caregivers are doing the best that they can, and the early mistakes they make are often the result of inexperience or a lack of knowledge. You may want your physician or another trusted individual to intervene on your behalf.

Elyse was a baker in a small city bakery. She had been married for fifteen years and was raising four children, two boys and two girls. When she was driving home from work early one morning, she was hit by a drunk driver who had run a red light. Her mental faculties were not damaged, but she became a quadriplegic as a result of her injuries. She received a generous financial settlement, which enabled her to continue living at home with twenty-four-hour care. She remained alert and competent, and insisted on continuing to make significant decisions about her children's upbringing. After her accident, however, three of her teenage children began to view their mother as "a typical quadriplegic" whose opinions were not important, and who no longer had authority over them. With the support of her husband, she let her children know in no uncertain terms that she was still their mother — and still in charge. She had just as much importance and authority as before the accident, and they were damn well going to respect it. Elyse's stern words and resolve convinced her children that their mother was still an able and devoted parent.

Their admiration for her increased, and they marvelled at her efforts to remain active and psychologically independent. It is essential for anyone with a disability to speak out, so that their role in their family or any other setting does not diminish.

Escape and Avoidance

Some of your close friends and family members may have difficulty coping with your disability. They may lack the emotional maturity, at least for an initial period of time, to provide you with the support you need. Some people may shy away from visiting, and family members may try to be out of the house as much as possible. This form of avoidance is known as escape.

You may have to give these people some time to re-evaluate their relationship and their obligations to you. They will often be able to reassess their roles and expectations, and then provide you with what you need. Try to allow time for them to adjust, even though they are making a difficult period even harder for you. Although you have a right to be angry, try to welcome them back with open arms when they are willing and able to help you. Family members should have the opportunity to discuss their concerns with each other and with professionals who can provide the information, education, and support that may permit them to cope more effectively with unforeseen and unanticipated feelings.

Sarah was a single woman in her mid-twenties who worked as a computer programmer. She sustained a head injury after tripping and falling down her stairs. Although the fall did not damage her intellectual capacity, it led to a severe stutter, which made her very difficult to understand. Sarah's speech impediment made many of her family members and friends uncomfortable. Some people would interrupt her and try to complete her sentences, and others would make excuses and try to avoid her company. In fact, she lost friends who did not want to make the effort to accommodate her condition. Fortunately, Sarah decided to take a proactive approach to her disability. She joined a support group for people who stuttered, where she learned strategies to help her communicate. She let her friends know that cutting her off in mid-sentence was hurtful and inappropriate, and she explained the strategies that enabled them all to feel comfortable. She maintained most of her relationships, and eventually married a man who was completely comfortable with her disability. He had the benefit of knowing how she felt, as they had met each other at the support group. People who felt comfortable with Sarah helped her to feel comfortable with herself.

Isolation

Some people with disabilities are unable to enjoy all of the activities they had engaged in prior to the onset of their condition. Others lose contact with their friends and family. I knew one man who was an active member of our community. He had terminal cancer, and had only a short time to live. Sadly, few of his friends visited him when he was in the hospital, and he became very upset. One day, he asked for a pen and notepaper. He wrote letters to all of his friends. The letters read: "I am dying today. What are you doing?" His gesture expressed the rage many people feel when their disability leads to isolation.

If people distance themselves from a friend or family member who has experienced a serious disability or terminal illness, it is not because they no longer care, but because they feel awkward or unsure how to respond appropriately. In other cases, partners are overwhelmed by their responsibilities, and are unwilling or unable to carry them out. Some friends and relatives will always be there for you, but others will not. If you are honest and let the people you care about know exactly how you feel, either in conversation or by correspondence, you will often be pleasantly surprised at how well they respond.

Violation of Privacy

Often, people with disabilities are not treated with respect. Family members and caregivers may feel that it is okay to violate your privacy in a way they never would have before. For example, when people with disabilities try to initiate intimate relationships, they are not always afforded the privacy to which they are entitled. This loss of privacy is particularly pronounced in an institutional setting, where caregivers feel they are responsible for residents at all times, and are reluctant to allow members of the opposite sex to be alone together. Demand your privacy in such a scenario.

Most caregivers will not intrude on your privacy out of ill will, but do it because they feel a responsibility to make sure that you are okay. Caregivers may hover at all hours, enter rooms at inappropriate times, and not leave you with any time to yourself. This problem can usually be resolved by a clear discussion of your concerns. It may be appropriate to acquire an alarm-like device that can be used to alert people when you are in need. In this way, both the giver and the receiver of care can have their needs addressed.

Loss of Sense of Adulthood

Some caregivers treat their adult patients as children. Many people become angry when caregivers treat them in this manner. Caregivers can be overprotective and insensitive, and can fail to realize that they are working with a mature adult who should never be talked down to or ignored. Professional caregivers should ask permission before referring to a client by his first name, and they should treat their clients as equals. If caregivers invade your privacy, tell them their behaviour is unacceptable.

People who reside in nursing homes are routinely addressed by their first names by strangers who are many years their junior. They are also talked down to, and their opinions and concerns are discounted. Some staff and administration will not listen to clients' complaints. The intervention and constant vigilance of family members and friends can ensure that these individuals are treated with compassion, respect, and dignity.

Anger

Some of your closest family members may express anger or disappointment in you because of your disability. In fact, many individuals are accused of being responsible for their own problems. Family members may also not want to be involved in this unexpected experience. They may feel that the new requirements of caregiving have limited their opportunities, and that they are uncomfortable with the prospect of assuming the responsibility. Anger sometimes indicates that an individual is self-centred and concerned only with his own welfare. In other situations, anger can result from feelings of frustration or a lack of control. Anger may also result if a caregiver does not receive the warmth and support that she used to receive from her partner. In extreme cases, anger may lead to physical or emotional abuse.

Linda was a seventeen-year-old high-school student. She was riding double with her boyfriend on his motorcycle when they were sideswiped by a motorist who was talking on his cellular phone. Linda was seriously injured. She lost the use of her right arm, and her right leg was severely incapacitated. After a lengthy stay in the hospital, she had been at home for three weeks when her parents began to criticize her stupidity for riding on the motor-cycle. They claimed that she was responsible for her injuries, and complained that they were going to be tied down for the rest of their lives because of her "inconsiderate behaviour." During this time, Linda was waging a courageous battle to be as independent as possible. Her parents' comments were hurtful and caused depression that required clinical treatment. Unfortunately, Linda's parents increased their verbal attacks, which in turn increased her depression. Linda was in considerable physical pain, and the emotional impact of her parents' anger set back her rehabilitation. She eventually moved out of her home to get away from this situation, and she continued her rehabilitation on her own. She overcame her injuries, and was self-sufficient and independent. She was an A student at a local university, where she earned a master's degree in social work, and entered a career in community organization. Her parents' anger was a barrier that she had to overcome before she could achieve success.

Support groups can help caregivers cope more effectively. These groups provide a sympathetic ear, caregiving expertise, and information about resources. Although a disability may render one's spouse temporarily dependent, the loss of balance in the relationship can be overcome through adaptation and rehabilitation. Many relationships emerge from disability stronger than they were before. If support is not available, however, individuals may feel so much frustration that they are unable to cope, and the relationship may come to an end.

FAMILY BREAKDOWN

Disability can place significant stresses on a family. If the tensions that are introduced are not managed properly, personal conflicts can be exacerbated and some relationships may end. A spouse or partner may feel that they are not obliged to bear the new responsibilities brought about by disability. If the partner without a disability leaves, there are several alternatives.

A relationship that ends because of a disability is, in many respects, the same as any relationship that ends. You have to focus on moving on and rebuilding your life. Take care of your immediate physical and emotional needs. If you have a disability for which you require day-to-day assistance, it may be necessary to hire a part-time or full-time caregiver. You may also consider moving in with other members of your family, or moving into a supported-living environment. If depression results from the severing of a serious relationship, professional counselling may be a good idea. If a spouse leaves, you may also have legal recourse to cover the costs of care, and may be in the position to receive a favourable divorce settlement.

CONCLUSION

Your family is usually the first source that you will turn to in times of need. The support of your loved ones will be a vital ingredient in the successful struggle against disability. The more people that you can draw on for support, the better. A group of friends with whom you can discuss your feelings, fears, choices, and hopes can make it much easier to cope. No matter how large your circle of friends, you will still encounter some tough times. However, your family and friends can help you to recognize the danger signs of negative coping, and take immediate action to address any difficulties that may arise. In this chapter we have discussed the strategies that will enable you and your family to identify and overcome the challenges that disability can pose. Now we turn to the steps you can take to make your living arrangements disability-friendly.

Chapter 3

Disability and the Home

INTRODUCTION

When I was young, my parents were told to put me in an institution. Doctors, friends, and family members told them that my care would be too difficult, that I was never going to accomplish anything, and that they "can always have more kids." I was very fortunate that they rejected this advice, and I was raised in a warm, supportive atmosphere where I was loved, encouraged, and stimulated. These surroundings helped me develop self-confidence, self-esteem, and the desire to succeed.

Where we live plays a central role in shaping our quality of life. Our home is a place where we can retain our identity and some control over our own lives. But disability may necessitate your making changes to your living arrangements, including renovations to increase accessibility, installing assistive technology, and hiring support staff. Most people with disabilities want to continue living at home, and indeed this is usually the most desirable alternative. Sometimes, however, the new challenges brought on by disability will require a change in residence on a temporary or permanent basis.

There are several residential options for people with disabilities. When choosing one of these options, you should always be trying to maximize your quality of life. This chapter outlines the positives and negatives of each arrangement, and will help you to make the appropriate choice in the event of a disability.

Where you live determines who you interact with, the activities you participate in, your work opportunities, and even your diet. People with disabilities enjoy many things that the world has to offer, but remaining active can be difficult for those who live in an isolated or restricted environment. When you are looking at making changes to your living arrangements in response to disability, the least restrictive alternative is usually the best.

HOUSING OPTIONS

Living at Home

Home is usually the most positive environment for anyone who has a disability. The family home allows the maximum possible level of freedom and integration, and in general, people who live at home usually enjoy a superior quality of life. Living with your family, or on your own, or with the support of a full-time caregiver, provides greater independence and inclusiveness than can be achieved in other settings.

The Benefits of Living at Home

- In the home, you are surrounded by family and friends who provide you with love, encouragement, and security.

Friends and family can become your most important allies in living with and overcoming disability.

- Residing at home improves your ability to maintain relationships with friends and relatives. People will always feel more comfortable visiting you in a familiar setting than in an institutional environment.

- Living at home allows you more freedom to be involved in social and recreational activities. You can usually have open access to a telephone and the Internet, so you need never be "alone." You can watch TV or listen to music free of restrictions. When you live at home you can keep your own hours, and you are not required to conform to a pre-set schedule for meals, activities, or bedtimes.

- Most homes can be adapted to accommodate alternative working arrangements. An increasing number of individuals continue to work after serious disabilities through the use of computers and other assistive technologies, including the Internet. It is easier to establish a new occupation when you have complete freedom over the design of your home and the hours that you work.

- Living at home allows you to continue eating what you want, with the people you want, rather than eating a set menu of mass-produced, institutional meals in the company of strangers. Although this may seem unimportant, the enjoyment of meals is something that people in institutional settings genuinely miss.

- Living with your family can have other benefits. Your family members are the ones who are most concerned with your welfare, and they will constantly motivate you to perform your exercises and rehabilitation program. When your family members are closely involved, they can push you to the peak of your ability.

- Support and respite services are often available from local governments, or private agencies, and volunteer, support, advocacy, and service groups can make home care easier.
- The cost of your care, although expensive, can be more reasonable at home than in an institution.

The Drawbacks of Home Care

Although home care provides many benefits, it can also create a number of social, emotional, and financial problems.

- The specialized care, therapy, educational services, and equipment that are available in an institutional environment cannot always be arranged in a home setting.
- Home care is a lot of work. The responsibility of caring for a family member can be onerous, and the requirements of care frequently cause physical strain and injury to caregivers. Lifting, bathing, dressing, transporting, and other tasks can place a heavy burden on someone who does not have the proper support or physical strength. For example, wives who take care of their husbands are highly susceptible to back injuries, from the strain of providing physical care.
- The strain on family members who act as caregivers can lead to emotional problems such as stress, burnout, alcoholism, and depression. Caregivers are especially vulnerable if they do not have access to adequate support services.
- Because of the cost, it can be difficult, if not impossible, to provide and maintain all of the specialized equipment you may need (from ramps and respirators to computer technology). It may also be prohibitively expensive to make the necessary renovations to your home.

Making the Most of Home Care

Extensive preparations are essential for home care to be effective. By consulting with the same doctors, support groups, and professionals who helped to educate you about disability, you can find out exactly what you will need to provide effective care. If you are planning for the care of a loved one, it is crucial that you take their wishes into account. If everyone works together, potential conflicts can be avoided.

Charlie

Charlie was a retired mailman who lived in Albany, New York. He spent his retirement with his wife, Anne, golfing, travelling, and visiting grandchildren. Five years after he retired, he began to have difficulty speaking and walking, and his co-ordination began to deteriorate. After consulting with a specialist, he was diagnosed with Parkinson's disease and it was recommended that he use a wheelchair. Charlie and Anne had lived in the same three-bedroom home for more than forty years. They had an emotional attachment to the home where their children had grown up, and did not want to leave. It was an older house, however, and was not wheelchair accessible. They looked into renting an apartment that was accessible, but found it was too expensive. They decided to modify their home to accommodate Charlie's disability.

On the recommendation of their physician, they had a district health worker and an expert in barrier-free design visit their home. They determined that Charlie and Anne would need a ramp to the front door, and that the entrances to every room would have to be widened to accommodate the chair. The bathroom also required extensive renovations, including the installation of a shower stall so Charlie could remain in his chair in the shower. Support bars, larger light switches, lower sinks, and lower shelves and counters had to be installed to make the home completely accessible. The renovation costs would probably exceed $20,000, money they did not have. Happily, Charlie had been a member of the Kiwanis Club for many years, and when they heard about his problems they arranged to have all of the labour contributed by volunteers. Charlie and Anne still had to pay for the raw materials, but even these were provided at wholesale price. The total cost they had to bear was $6,200. The changes were made, and they were able to continue enjoying life at home.

Making Your Home Disability-Friendly

Advance preparation for disability can save you from having to make expensive renovations later on. If possible, take accessibility issues into account when buying or renting a home. For maximum accessibility, a home should have all of its rooms on the same level and outside entrances should be as close as possible to street level. In this respect, apartment dwellers often have an advantage. If you have an older residence, or if your home has more than one floor, it is unlikely that it will have these attributes. However, there are several other features that are important:

- stairways wide enough to accommodate a chair lift;
- sufficient room on the property to add a bedroom and bathroom to the main floor to aid accessibility or accommodate a parent or caregiver;
- proximity to public transportation, medical care, shopping, and entertainment facilities.

Renovations and Technological Support

The renovations you make to your home will vary according to the nature of your disability. If you are renovating to accommodate a disability, some construction firms may be willing to provide discounts. Service clubs, religious groups, and disability organizations will also often provide personnel and contributions, which can alleviate some of your expenses. Some financial institutions have also been known to provide lower-interest loans for disability-related renovations.

For individuals who have rheumatism, arthritis, Parkinson's, and similar conditions, climbing stairs, opening doors, using a can opener — what we consider to be the most basic of activities — can become painful and difficult, and even impossible. Charlie was able to enjoy independent living in a barrier-free environment that was specially adapted to his needs. A family friend with rheumatoid arthritis also had to adapt her apartment so she could continue to live there. She installed doors that opened by remote control to supplement the standard grab bars and special handles. She also invested in specialized technology — including large-handled knives, forks, and can openers — that made basic tasks much easier. Her occupational therapist assessed the assistive devices that she would find most useful, and she picked up other suggestions from members of her support group.

The Family Residence with In-Home Support

Harvey was a dentist in his early fifties who had a severe stroke as a result of an infected heart valve. He was unable to speak following the stroke, and he could move only his left leg. He did not want to live in an institution, but his wife was unable to provide the necessary care. Fortunately, he had an insurance plan that covered the cost of caregivers in the event of a disabling condition. This enabled him to arrange twenty-four-hour, in-home care.

He remained involved with his friends, family, and community, regained the ability to communicate, and after several months of therapy gained the strength to move his own wheelchair. He reads books (with a caregiver to turn the page), and enjoys watching television, taking day trips in local parks, and eating out at fine restaurants. He controls his own schedule and diet, and enjoys the freedom of living at home.

Like Harvey, many people are able to continue living at home with the assistance of support personnel, an arrangement that has many advantages:

- It allows you to reap all the benefits of living at home, even if you require intensive, constant, and specialized supervision and care.
- Outside caregivers ease the burden on and responsibilities of family members, allowing them greater independence and more time to "recharge their batteries." This will make the time that they commit to care more productive.
- Paying for outside support while living at home is usually cheaper than institutional living, and allows for a quality of life that can seldom be duplicated in an institution.
- When family members work side by side with professional caregivers, a high level of care is assured. As a result, the chances for inadequate treatment or abuse are significantly diminished.

If it is possible, living in one's community is preferable to living in an institutional setting. Even if you require round-the-clock supervision, it is better to receive it at home.

Support and Incentives to Home Care

Some government agencies provide incentives that encourage individuals to care for family members within the home. These incentives even cover financial aid for renovations, including the installation of ramps, widened doors, specialized washroom equipment, and elevators.

The costs of full- or part-time staff may also be augmented by grants. Nurses, physiotherapists, and other caregivers may be paid for in part by assistance from municipal, state, or provincial governments. You also have the option of purchasing an insurance policy to cover these extra costs. If you lack adequate coverage, or if the support that is available is insufficient, service groups, religious organizations, or personnel from colleges or universities may provide excellent volunteer support. Support groups are also indispensable in these endeavours.

PART-TIME INSTITUTIONAL CARE

If a person loses a limb or encounters another type of serious disability, it may be difficult for her to adjust, especially in the short term. It is often productive for these individuals to attend an institution for an initial period of rehabilitation. Institutions can provide intensive therapy and instruction in the best self-help techniques, which can ease the adjustment to disability.

This type of mixed care is best for people with significant disabilities who are still able to live at home, but who also require intensive therapy. Institutions that cater to part-time residents or out-patients frequently offer services to accommodate their clients' needs, such as day-care services and flexible access to institutional resources, in addition to therapy, counselling, and recreation.

An institution will also provide individuals with a transition period, during which they can gain inspiration and encouragement from seeing other people who face similar challenges. Sometimes, these adjustment periods can even be shortened by a sense of competition. Said one thirty-year-old amputee, on witnessing a seventy-eight-year-old walking around on an artificial leg, "If that old bastard can do it, so can I!" Being in an environment where you can see how other people in the same boat are coping can have a positive effect on your own ability to adjust.

Sandra was a twenty-two-year-old college student from New York who planned on being a model. She was working as a waitress in a restaurant, and sustained a severe spinal injury when she was hit by a stray bullet during an attempted robbery. As a result of the injury, she lost the use of both legs and had partial upper-body paralysis. When the injury occurred, she was living at home with her parents. But she moved into an institution after her hospital stay because her parents were unable to provide the level of care and rehabilitation she needed. The rehabilitation centre had specially trained personnel and equipment, and focused on intensive daily therapy. Sandra lived in the rehab centre for slightly less than a year, during which time she was able to regain the use of her hands and arms, and learn the living skills necessary to become independent. She enrolled in a university social work program and is well on her way to building a successful career. For Sandra and others like her, institutions provide intensive training that is not available in any other setting.

Anything that can improve the rate or extent of your recovery or adjustment is beneficial. Simply determine what mixture will bring the most positive results. If the intensive therapy that you require can be provided only in an institutional setting, then it is in your interests to pursue it, to achieve the greater goal of long-term independence. Many institutions are more flexible than in the past, and encourage their patients to take weekends and holidays with friends and family whenever possible.

The amount of time spent in an institution will depend on the individual's physical needs and her motivation. For many, part-time care is the best choice because it allows patients access to specialized resources, while they still reap the benefits of the family environment.

When Is Part-Time Institutional Care Appropriate?

Part-time institutional care is advantageous for those who have had strokes or head injuries, and who must endure long and difficult rehabilitative and educational programs to regain their capacities. It may also be a viable option for people in the early stages of Alzheimer's disease, because it ensures that they are involved in specialized activities that focus on maintaining their mental abilities for as long as possible. Time spent in the facility also provides relief for those members of the family who ordinarily provide care.

Condition-specific institutions provide specialized therapy for people experiencing the same condition. For example, when an individual loses her hearing or sight, she can enter a short-term facility where she can learn sign language or how to read Braille. This narrow focus can be extremely effective.

Part-time institutional care not only stimulates the patient, but also eventually provides for a better quality of life than other living arrangements. It is less expensive than full-time institutional care.

INDEPENDENT LIVING CENTRES (ILCs)

Before the 1970s, there were few places where people with disabilities could live on their own that took their personal needs into account. In the past three decades, however, independent living centres (ILCs) have filled this vacuum. Independent living centres provide educational, recreational, and social programs specially tailored to their residents' needs. These apartment or homestyle facilities are supervised, and provide the advantages of independence within a protective environment. Some independent living centres are government subsidized, and many also receive support from service clubs and other organizations. Some residents are self-supporting and contribute to the cost of their own housing. Most residents view the ILC not as an institution, but as a residence in which they can maximize their opportunities, just like any other apartment or boarding-house. They are proud to be there.

Eric

Eric was a steelworker in Pittsburgh who had a wife and a son. He enjoyed watching the Steelers, was active in his local church, and was a little-league baseball coach. He decided to have surgery on his back to relieve severe chronic pain caused by the heavy lifting his job required. The surgery went wrong, leaving Eric in a very weak state and in even worse pain. He was no longer able to work, and he went on a disability pension. He tried living at home, but his wife was unable to provide the level of care he required. He needed help getting in and out of bed, negotiating stairs, using the bathroom, and performing many other tasks. On bad days, he was unable to feed himself. He and his wife couldn't afford attendant care.

Eric did not want to live in an institution. Fortunately, the family clergyman was aware of a new independent living centre that had just opened. Eric went for an interview and to examine the ILC. He found that the residents received a high level of care, with access to chiropractors and other medical specialists. Through a residents' council, residents were able to make their own decisions about curfews, meals, recreation, and anything else of importance. All thirty-seven residents in the ILC voted on decisions affecting their treatment and care. Eric could leave to visit his family whenever he wanted, and he was able to have visitors at any time. In addition, the facility was new and contained a therapy pool, a gym, a pool table, and a home-entertainment system. There was a room set aside for parties and other private family gatherings. Although the facility was not home, it provided the support Eric required. He remains happily married, and continues to live in the ILC.

The Benefits of Independent Living Centres

- ILCs provide people with disabilities with greater control over their living conditions. Unlike some families, which exclude members with disabilities from the decision-making process, ILCs provide everyone with the opportunity to participate.
- Residents' councils are often established to allow residents to participate in the determination of the policies that govern their "community living." Through these councils, residents are able to direct caregivers on how to perform their duties. Councils also schedule entertainment and recreational programs, set out resident responsibilities, arrange transportation, select medical and para-medical personnel, and even choose menus. This high level of responsibility and independence is a very effective means of building residents' self-esteem and maintaining or developing their independent living skills.
- ILCs provide a greater opportunity for privacy than many family homes.
- ILCs provide the opportunity to develop new friendships. They also provide an open social atmosphere that can lead to intimate relationships.

- The supervision in these centres is provided by individuals who are trained to meet the residents' needs.
- ILCs protect people with disabilities from becoming dependent on family members or caregivers. ILCs are based on the principle of "safe independence," which allows as much individual freedom as possible without sacrificing safety and security.
- ILCs usually cost less than institutions. In fact, because the housing units are operated as non-profit accommodations, the cost is often less than that of a regular apartment of a similar size and location.

The Drawbacks of Independent Living Centres

- Because the residents' councils define policies, some people are forced to endure decisions and rules with which they do not agree. Democratic decision-making tends to be effective, but if votes consistently go against your wishes, this style of living can become increasingly irritating and unpleasant.
- Because most people move into ILCs on their own, their roommates are initially strangers, and this can lead to discomfort. Although a sense of community will usually develop quickly among residents, some individuals find the adjustment difficult, while others are uncomfortable with or dislike their roommates or fellow residents.
- In an ILC, an individual can be separated from her family and friends. This can have a negative impact on motivation and personal comfort, especially in the initial transition period.

How to Get the Most Out of an Independent Living Centre

Because the residents' councils determine the policies for each ILC, active participation in the decision-making process is the best way to ensure a positive experience. Before entering an ILC, you should read all of the information provided and visit the centre to ensure that you are compatible with the other residents and the staff.

What If There Are No ILCs in My Area?

Many smaller communities do not have ILCs. To counter this, some individuals with disabilities have brought together financial supporters, social workers, and caregivers. These groups then purchase, lease, or rent an apartment or home, renovate it, and staff it to duplicate the programs available in independent living centres, albeit on a smaller scale. These individualized residences provide all of the benefits of traditional ILCs.

INSTITUTIONAL CARE

Institutional care is chosen as a last resort, only when it becomes almost impossible to care for an individual at home. People in the late stages of Alzheimer's, Parkinson's disease, Lou Gehrig's disease, and other degenerative conditions are among the most common residents of institutions. Even though an institution may be the "last stop" for many, that does not mean it is a place devoid of life. On the contrary, people in these difficult situations benefit most from the intensity and specialization of high-quality institutional care.

The Benefits of Full-Time Institutional Care

- The institution offers specialized equipment; physical, occupational, and drug therapy; social activities; and access to personnel and programs that may not be available in other settings.
- Institutions are able to provide care for people with the most serious of disabilities, those whose requirements may be beyond that which can be provided in the family home. Some staffs include specialists in pain management, who are able to alleviate the suffering of patients with severe illnesses through the most efficient and modern methods and equipment.
- Institutions also provide intensive counselling and support to their patients. Most institutions have links to the clergy, as well as to grief counsellors, who are sensitive to the needs of people in distress.
- A state or non-profit institution can provide a place for adults who simply cannot afford or cannot cope with home care.

The Drawbacks of Full-Time Institutional Care

- Institutional care cannot duplicate the strong emotional ties that are maintained in the family home. An institutional resident is separated from his friends and family, and is thus highly susceptible to loneliness.
- Some institutions are understaffed, leading to inadequate services, programs, and care. In addition, care is frequently very impersonal.
- Some of the personnel may be underqualified, or unqualified, for the tasks they perform. In medical emergencies,

for example, unqualified staff are less likely to respond appropriately. This can result in severe injury and even the loss of life.

- Medications are often given out on institutional, rather than individual, schedules. Some institutions have the flexibility to allow those residents who are able to manage their own medication or follow a SAM (self-administered medication) program.
- Institutions can be very expensive.
- Social, psychological, physical, and sexual abuse can occur.
- If the institution does not provide a warm and supportive environment, a patient may withdraw, becoming unresponsive or, in some cases, violent. As a result, patients are sometimes restrained or overmedicated instead of being treated in a more humane manner. In one case, an individual with psychiatric difficulties who was screaming repeatedly from the pain of a twisted bowel was put in a strait-jacket by staff members who thought he was just "acting out." This was an isolated incident, but institutions can make it difficult, if not impossible, for patients to convey the fact that they are in physical distress.

How Do I Select the Best Institution?

The best way to choose a high-quality institution is through careful research. Social services agencies and support groups who have worked closely with an institution can give you an idea of its strengths and weaknesses. Visiting the facility to evaluate the surroundings and talk to staff members can help provide a complete picture. Talking to residents and their family members to gauge their level of satisfaction with the care provided can also help you make a decision. Many of these facilities encourage prospective clients to visit. Take them up on the offer.

Facilities that are maintained by ethnic and religious groups are often superior to privately run institutions. These groups are usually concerned with preserving the highest possible quality of life, rather than with earning a profit. Religious and ethnic groups constantly work to improve their residents' surroundings, and their primary focus is their members' quality of life. The most expensive private facilities usually provide a high level of care, although this can sometimes cost between $6,000 and $10,000 a month. Not-for-profit facilities, on the other hand, can sometimes provide comparable or superior care at a significantly lower price.

Making the Most of the Institutional Experience

Outside the home, care for people with disabilities is usually not perfect. It's expensive, and the level of care may still be less than what is necessary or acceptable. Family members and other volunteers must be on their guard to ensure that their loved ones receive the care and attention to which they are entitled.

Most of these facilities are inspected by government officials. During inspections the institutions must meet all of the regulatory standards and provide all of the benefits that they have advertised. Some institutions, however, have been known to decrease their level of care substantially between inspections. A family member's constant involvement in a loved one's care is vital to ensuring that the level of service is maintained. Talking to other families of residents to identify and solve problems is also very important. If the institution is providing your loved one with substandard care, it is likely that he is not the only one. Many institutional residents are not cognitively impaired; they have the ability to identify areas of concern, yet do not have the power to make the administration act on their concerns. The existence of a residents' council that has real decision-making power and can address these concerns indicates that a facility provides quality care.

Jeremy

Jeremy was a landscape architect who retired at sixty-five and lived at home with his wife, Irene. In his early seventies, he started becoming absent-minded and forgetful. He was diagnosed with Alzheimer's disease, which was not a surprise, as his two older sisters had experienced the same condition. Irene cared for him at home for more than ten years, but by the time he reached his early eighties, he required a high level of nursing care that his wife could no longer provide. The family located a nursing home with a good reputation, in which Jeremy would be adequately cared for.

Irene soon discovered, however, that the program of care the nursing home advertised differed substantially from what was actually delivered. She noticed that her husband's clothing was frequently soiled, and that he appeared to be underfed and in need of social stimulation. Irene started pressuring the institution's administration on her husband's behalf, demanding that he be properly fed and stimulated, both physically and socially. She even hired an additional attendant to work with him for four hours every day and to take care of all his needs. The staff at the institution recognized that Irene would never accept second-rate care for her husband, and improved their efforts. Soon other families began to follow her example, and together they improved the overall level of care within the institution.

HOSPICES

A hospice is a living environment for people with terminal conditions that eases the transition of their final days. Hospices are peaceful environments that focus on minimizing the physical and emotional pain of their residents. Professional counsellors offer support, pain management, and drug therapy which allows people to die with dignity and with a minimum amount of pain.

Terry

Terry was a twenty-seven-year-old musician from Toronto. He was a hemophiliac who contracted AIDS through a blood transfusion in the mid-1980s. With a combination of drugs, he was able to fight the infection for five years, but he eventually contracted both tuberculosis and a severe infection from cuts he sustained in a car accident. He became very weak and checked into a hospital. Doctors told him that he had only one or two months to live, but that by taking extraordinary measures they could perhaps double this time. Terry spent three weeks in the hospital before he decided that he had had enough of the invasive and painful treatments, and of staff who treated him like "a leper" because of his terminal condition. He decided to move to a local hospice. The caregivers at the hospice were experts in pain management, and focused on providing care, compassion, and support, rather than on prolonging life. The staff members were honest and sincere, and did not treat the fact that he was going to die as a personal "failure." For Terry, the most important thing was that the staff members knew how to talk to him. They were completely at ease with terminal patients, and they helped him feel at peace. His friends and family were free to visit at any time, unlike the restricted visiting hours of the hospital, and when he died he was surrounded by loved ones. Before he died, Terry told me that the hospice had enriched his last days and helped him die in peace.

CONCLUSION

It is important for everyone to live in an environment in which they feel comfortable and safe. If you are living with a disability you should strive to maintain your level of independence and privacy, and remain close to your friends and favourite activities. If you require a high level of care, however, you may have to yield a portion of your freedom in order to maintain access to the necessary care. No matter where you are living, you should always be treated with respect and courtesy. You can tailor any living arrangement to meet your needs at home or in the workplace. We will now look at how people with disabilities can succeed in the working world.

Chapter

4

Disability and Work

INTRODUCTION

When I was going to school, many people, from grade school teachers to university professors, told me that I was never going to be able to support myself, that I was never going to be able to hold a job. People thought that because of my cerebral palsy, no one would hire me, and even if I was hired, they thought that I couldn't do a good job. I have been proving them wrong for the last thirty-two years.

Inaccessible workplaces, prejudicial hiring, and biased human resource policies have made it difficult for people with disabilities to gain access to the labour force. In addition, there is a widespread misconception that people with disabilities are lazy or incapable of working. Nothing could be further from the truth. Most people with disabilities are highly motivated and want to work. The percentage of people with disabilities who participate in the workforce is continually increasing — from 1986–1991, the participation rate for people with disabilities grew from 49 percent to 56 percent. Although this improvement is rapid, the participation rate for people without disabilities is approximately 80 percent.

Legislation, consciousness raising, and activism by disability groups have all helped to remove these barriers and create opportunities, but the work is ongoing. Studies have found that the existence of a disability is not the primary determinant of employment. A worker's education, skills, motivation, and environment are most important. People with disabilities that many would consider severe and limiting continue to accomplish amazing things.

Christopher Reeve

Christopher Reeve first became famous as the star of the Superman movies. He has acted in numerous movies, and was an outspoken activist for the arts and for the homeless. He was competing in a show jumping competition when he was thrown off his horse and severely injured. He became quadriplegic, paralysed from the neck down. Reeve has gone through a grueling rehabilitation program, and regained his ability to speak and breathe on his own. He has also renewed his activist efforts speaking on behalf of spinal-cord research and people with disabilities. Although many people would have believed it impossible, Reeve is also continuing his career in the entertainment industry. Recently he starred in, directed, and produced a remake of the Alfred Hitchcock thriller *Rear Window*. Christopher Reeve serves as an inspirational role model for people who encounter serious disabilities.

OBSTACLES IN THE WORKPLACE

Where you work and what you do are key components of your identity. What you accomplish through work builds and maintains your self-esteem, and provides concrete achievements in which you can take pride. Disability can prevent you from working on a temporary or permanent basis. People who couldn't work because of their disability have told me that the loss of self-esteem and the financial pressures brought on by their inability to work were the worst consequences of their disability. Being unable to work can destroy your independence.

People with disabilities have the highest rates of unemployment and underemployment of any group in society. The unemployment rate for people with disabilities is estimated at more than 80 percent. Even when these people have the skills to perform a job, they are often denied proper consideration because it is assumed by many that employees without disabilities will be able to do a better job, or that the employee with a disability will be incompetent, unreliable, or expensive to accommodate. As a result, it can be very difficult for people with disabilities to gain entry-level positions or to move up in the workplace. In actuality, workers with disabilities are among the most highly motivated in any workforce, and are able to carry out their duties effectively.

Although the legal system prohibits discrimination on the basis of disability, it is often very difficult to prove that a disability has been an influential factor in hiring and promotion decisions. Legal clinics and support groups often provide assistance for people with special needs, and will sometimes be able to help them get their needs addressed. But in ambiguous situations, it is often better to avoid legal action because of the high costs involved and the difficulty in proving discrimination. If, however, you experience clear-cut discrimination on the basis of your disability, then you should not hesitate in pursuing legal redress.

RETURNING TO WORK TOO QUICKLY

Sometimes workers with disabilities encounter other, non-legal difficulties that need to be resolved. Most people who experience disability want to return to work as soon as possible. They are committed to their jobs and are bored with inactivity. Many of them also fear being unable to return to work, or being left without sufficient income. As a result, they may be inclined to return to work even though they are not physically ready. Many people are unaware of their limitations until they get back to the workplace, where they may discover that they cannot cope.

Returning to work before you are physically able poses several problems:

1. You may not be able to requalify for short- or long-term disability benefits, depending on the coverage offered by your plan.
2. An employer may feel that your disability will require increased time off and other support, and may pass you over for promotion, offer early retirement, or demote you.
3. An employer may be reluctant to continue the terms of employment if he believes that you can no longer effectively perform your duties.
4. Employers and insurers may begin to doubt the legitimacy of your disability, depriving you of opportunities and benefits.

For these reasons, it is important to have a realistic sense of what you can do at any given time. Strive to rehabilitate as quickly as possible, but resist the temptation to return to work before you are ready.

The Benefits of a Graduated Work-Return Program

One of the best ways for an employee to ease the return to work following a major disability is to work with her employer to develop a graduated work-return program. A graduated work-return program allows the employee to acclimatize herself once again to the demands of the working environment by returning to work on a part-time basis. This enables her to develop the physical and mental endurance that will allow her to perform her job successfully. Most employers will be receptive to this type of program, which gives individuals every opportunity to return to work. This policy also helps to maintain and even increase morale in the workplace, as other employees realize that they are valued and will be supported in times of hardship.

Sometimes an individual may find that although he is able to perform high-quality work, he does not have the stamina to resume all of his former responsibilities. In this scenario, an employee will often be able to negotiate a more flexible work schedule, or to work full time but on reduced hours. If employers can avoid the trouble and expense of hiring and training new staff, they will often be willing to do so.

I was unable to work for six months after my heart attack. Following my surgery in April, I recuperated until September, at which point I resumed teaching, at two-thirds of my previous workload. Initially, work was difficult and tiring, but I was able to carry out my teaching and research responsibilities successfully. Within a year, I had returned to teaching a full course load, but on a modified schedule. Instead of teaching three courses each semester for two semesters, I teach two courses each semester for three semesters. This flexibility enabled me and my employer to continue our mutually beneficial relationship.

CHANGING PROFESSIONS

Sometimes a disability will prevent you from resuming your previous occupation. If this occurs, it does not mean that you will be completely unable to work. Occupational therapists will assess your abilities and direct you into training programs for alternative employment. Some of the fields that people with disabilities most commonly enter are social work, counselling, computer science, consulting, teaching, call dispatching, marketing and telemarketing, clerical work, and banking. If you are faced with changing your profession as a result of disability, do not feel limited to these choices. People with disabilities can do anything!

Randy lived in Buffalo and drove a tractor-trailer from city to city in New York State. He would load and unload his own truck, and make adjustments to the tractor. When he was forty-seven, the discs in his back deteriorated significantly. This caused back pain so severe that he was unable to sit behind the wheel for extended periods of time, or to perform any maintenance work on his rig. Randy worked for a large international trucking company, and his long-term disability insurance provided him with income for five years, which enabled him to enrol in a training program for human-resource managers at a local college. He went to school for two years and did well in all of his classes. After graduation, he landed a job in human-resource management that paid him the same amount he made as a truck driver. Randy never anticipated having to change careers. Fortunately, his long-term disability insurance paid for his family's expenses and his education until he was able to establish a new career.

Technology, Employment, and Education

Increasingly, advanced computers and other assistive technologies are enabling people with even the most serious disabilities to gain expertise in a wide range of fields. Voice synthesizers, programs that read text out loud, cursors that respond to eye movements, and many other devices are available, allowing people with quadriplegia and other disabilities to communicate. The technologies are improving at an exponential rate. People who had difficulty communicating at more than a few words a minute several years ago can now communicate effectively through the use of technology.

Computers also provide people with disabilities access to educational opportunities that were not available only ten years ago. Correspondence courses can be done entirely by computer, all essays and assignments can be sent in by e-mail or fax, and the Internet provides a wealth of information for anyone who wants it. The prospects for retraining following a serious disability are also much better than ever before. Occupational therapists are experts in developing rehabilitation programs to get individuals back to work, or to retrain them for alternative employment.

WHAT HAPPENS IF YOU CAN'T WORK ANY MORE?

There are many individuals who love the responsibility, sense of achievement, and compensation provided by their employment. These people will often be reluctant to give up their jobs, even when the physical challenges are overwhelming. They make heroic efforts to try to fulfil their responsibilities, often in co-operation with their employers, who are inspired by the courage they demonstrate and go to great lengths to accommodate them. Unfortunately, however, there are times when people must finally relinquish their positions. When they can no longer perform their duties, their efforts to continue working inflict severe physical and psychological damage.

Ron

Ron worked as a manager of an office for many years. In his mid-thirties, he developed multiple sclerosis (a degenerative condition that causes fatigue and chronic pain, and curtails dexterity and mobility). He worked for six years after he was diagnosed, making constant adjustments as his condition deteriorated. He had a van specially adapted so he could drive it from his own wheelchair, and he had hand controls installed after he lost the ability to safely use the foot pedal and brakes. As he lost the dexterity in his fingers, he was given a verbally operated computer, which allowed him to continue his work. He gradually lost the ability to write, pick up the phone, drive, or use the public transportation system. He made valiant efforts to continue to perform his duties, but after five and a half years his productivity severely diminished, owing to the fatigue and pain associated with his condition. Although some drugs were helpful, it became clear that he could no longer continue. The organization he was with recognized his loyalty and supported his efforts, but towards the end of his sixth year working with MS, it became clear that he could no longer carry out his responsibilities. Ron had an emotional meeting with the CEO, during which they both agreed that it would be for the best if he stepped down. Ron had a disability plan that replaced a significant portion of his income, and he retired to focus on living with his MS.

Ron's employer was sympathetic and supportive, but also recognized that continued employment was impossible. The organization had made every effort to accommodate his disability. In other situations, employers may not be as understanding and may pressure you to retire. If you can no longer perform the duties of your job, your boss has the right to terminate employment. But if you can still work effectively, you should not be forced to leave.

If you find it difficult to work, discuss your problems openly with your superiors. You can try to find alternatives that will allow you to keep working (including being assigned alternative responsibilities). Also, take the time to learn about all of the benefits to which you are entitled.

CONCLUSION

Many people with disabilities can be successful in the job market if they are given the opportunity to work and reasonable accommodation. By choosing or building an environment that is suited to your needs, you will be able to flourish. Your skills and knowledge should determine your success in the workplace, not your disability. There are many strategies you can use to prevent an accident or disability from disrupting or ending your working life. All over the world people with disabilities are showing what they can achieve, and are eroding the prejudices of the past.

Advocacy: Getting What You Want and What You Need

INTRODUCTION

I have been an advocate all my life. I have stood up to be counted, shouted, yelled, persuaded, pleaded, sued, argued, and worked to get what I deserve. I have fought every step of the way, from grade school, through high school and university, and even all the way to the Supreme Court of Canada, to get people to accept me and accommodate my disability. In this chapter, I will share with you what I have learned about advocacy, so you, too, can become an effective advocate.

Advocacy is the art of getting what you need and what you deserve. It is an approach to problem-solving that will enable you to get the best available services and to contend effectively with disability. Advocacy is an indispensable tool that will help you get first-rate diagnoses, treatment, and care. The strategies of advocacy will help you manage all of the problems your disability may cause.

Advocacy is also an attitude. When people first experience disability, they often feel overwhelmed and may not know what to think or do. Instead of sitting back and passively hoping that everything will unfold for you, **you have to take control!** No matter what you are attempting to achieve, take the attitude that your needs (or the needs of your loved one) are more important than anything else, and that you will not be satisfied until your concerns are addressed.

When you are just starting out as an advocate, it can be difficult to put your own interests first. You may feel uncomfortable if your demands cause you to step on toes, offend someone, or appear selfish. Don't be afraid to act with a strong sense of self-interest. Advocacy is not mere egotism; advocacy is aimed at guaranteeing the quality of your care and your living conditions. When you participate in advocacy efforts, you may help others as well.

Traditionally, people with disabilities were expected to be quiet, deferential, and grateful for whatever benefits they were granted. This attitude prevented them from being treated fairly. Put aside any fears or reluctance you have about "rocking the boat" and become a strong advocate. You *can* take responsibility for getting what you need!

DIFFERENT KINDS OF ADVOCACY

Advocacy can range from personal efforts to get medical and hospital staff to be open and honest with you about your care to massive, nationwide efforts to enact legislation or change the constitution. No matter what level you are acting on, the same principles will apply.

Advocacy on the National Level

On the national level, advocacy efforts are marked by the co-operation of numerous different groups, massive fund-raising efforts, and the involvement of the local, state or provincial, and federal governments. These efforts can take several years from start to finish. For example, in the United States, activists began laying the groundwork for the Americans with Disabilities Act (ADA) in the mid-1970s. George Bush embraced the ADA during the 1988 presidential campaign, and disability groups and their allies across the country rallied to his support to have the act enshrined in the constitution. They focused on getting Bush elected so he could fulfil his promise. It is estimated that 4 million people with disabilities and their supporters changed their votes to support Bush. This massive change in voter intentions was estimated to have given President Bush 60 percent of his margin of victory. Once elected, George Bush followed through on his promise. Within two years of his election to office, the ADA was passed into law.

Case Study: Making Accessibility a Public Issue

Until the early 1980s, sidewalk curbs in most urban communities were not ramped. This made negotiating local neighbourhoods very difficult for people with mobility impairments, especially those who used wheelchairs. Few people or politicians were aware of the issue, because the need for accessibility was not publicized. When isolated activists did raise the issue, politicians were able to dismiss their concerns because of the high construction costs.

In the early 1980s, local disability groups across the continent began a consciousness-raising campaign aimed at alerting their fellow citizens and city counsellors to their needs. Activists marched, they wrote letters to politicians and businesspeople who could contribute funding, and they launched media campaigns to place their issues on the public agenda. They claimed that they were entitled to the same rights and privileges as other minorities. But they did not ask for hand-outs. They wanted access so they could participate in society and become taxpayers. They asked, "How can we get jobs if we can't even get to work? And even if we get to work, we can't get in the buildings!"

This message began to gain acceptance in the mid-1980s. Until that time, members of disability groups had tended to focus on the problems associated with their own particular condition. By banding together, they gained recognition and power and were able to use this new-found clout to have their communal issues addressed. The consciousness-raising efforts, when supported by legislation, forced communities to take action, making not only sidewalks, but also public buildings accessible.

Advocacy on the Local Level

Tens of thousands of effective advocacy campaigns have been launched on a local level. These initiatives have included lobbying by people with sight impairments for audio signals that would alert them when traffic lights had changed colour; people with mobility impairments pushing for access to public transportation; and people insisting on a greater say in their own medical care.

A number of seniors in Vancouver were very upset that public transportation was not accessible to the elderly, many of whom had a disability. The buses were not wheelchair-accessible, and many of the major transportation stops were not within walking distance of seniors' residences. This active group of senior citizens wrote letters to civic politicians and the provincial government detailing their concerns. They enlisted the support of organizations for the hearing- and sight-impaired and other disabilities, as well as service organizations. Spokespeople in the coalition made every effort to appear on local radio and TV stations to get their message out. As a result of these efforts, the Greater Vancouver regional government, with the support of the provincial government, created a transportation system for seniors with disabilities. Some buses were retrofitted and new, accessible buses were also purchased. In addition, seniors with disabilities were able to buy subsidized taxi coupons, which covered 50 percent of their fares.

THE DIFFERENT KINDS OF ADVOCATES

When you first encounter disability, you may not feel that you can be an effective advocate. With time, however, almost anyone can gain the skills, knowledge, and confidence to be successful. Even after you have gained experience advocating on your own behalf, you may find that there are some issues for which you require outside assistance. There are many varieties of advocates who can support your efforts and supply the skills and knowledge that you need. The list below identifies the nine main kinds of advocates and what they do. We then explain when each type of advocacy is appropriate.

Types of Advocates

Self-Advocate
Self-advocacy covers all efforts made by an individual on one's own behalf.

Designated Advocate
A designated advocate is a family member or other chosen individual who supports your advocacy efforts or advocates on your behalf until you are able to manage your own affairs.

Citizen Advocate
A citizen advocate is a volunteer who works to defend the rights and interests of a person with a disability. Citizen advocates can

act as designated advocates, and they can also provide physical and emotional support.

Case Manager

A case manager is a professional who provides you with the information you need to plan your own care. A case manager is an expert who can direct you to specialists and facilities, and can provide comprehensive information about your options.

Social Work–Sponsored Advocate

Social work–sponsored advocates are usually employed by community agencies, such as hospitals, community clinics, or community social-service offices. Social work–sponsored advocates will provide you with emotional support and help to ensure that you receive appropriate treatment.

Legal Advocates and Legal Clinics

If you are involved in a situation in which legal action becomes necessary, it is usually advisable to obtain advice from lawyers who specialize in human-rights cases or from legal-aid clinics that represent the needs of special-interest groups. A legal advocate will perform litigation or legal negotiations on your behalf.

Special Advocate

Special advocates are experts in one particular policy or treatment area. They will take action only in their area of expertise. If you have a problem or question in one of these areas, their help can be invaluable.

Advocacy Groups

Advocacy groups act as resource centres. They have specialists in many different aspects of disability. They serve as a clearinghouse for information, and will also take on and support selected advocacy efforts.

Social Action Groups
Social action groups focus on a wide range of civil- and human-rights issues. They further the integration and empowerment of people with special needs through financial support, and through support for disability-friendly political candidates and legislation.

When Self-Advocacy Is Appropriate

Almost anyone has the ability to become a successful advocate on his own behalf, but it takes confidence, dedication, education, and practice. You must always attempt to be the strongest voice speaking out on your own behalf. If you can be your own advocate, do so! Speaking with experienced advocates before you start can give you a good idea of where to begin.

Alvin
Alvin owned his own small business, an advertising firm. He lived with severe arthritis, which responded well to intensive therapy. His doctor advised Alvin that the best treatment for his condition was warm-water hydrotherapy, which would help maintain his dexterity and keep his joints relatively loose. Alvin did not have access to a private pool, however, and the municipal pools were heated to only 76°F (24°C), which is ideal for recreational swimming but unacceptable for warm-water hydrotherapy. Alvin belonged to an arthritis support group, which had other members who would benefit from similar therapy. He decided to put his background in advertising to work. First, he contacted other disability groups whose members could use hydrotherapy, and he enlisted their co-operation in developing a working coalition. Their goal was to gain access to

three or four public pools across the community, and have them heat the waters to 90°F (32°C) three days a week so the hydrotherapy would be effective. Next, they established a list of key contacts, which included directors and recreational supervisors of community pools, members of the parks department, local politicians, and members of the media. Alvin then designed a mass mailing, which was sent out to each of the key contacts and followed up by a phone call. At first, they met with resistance because no public pool wanted the extra expense of heating its facilities to the required level. The coalition reminded the recreation boards, however, that the people who were requesting this service were also taxpayers who were entitled to accessible exercise programs. After three months of negotiations, two community pools agreed to provide for the hydrotherapy three times a week, which was sufficient to meet the needs of Alvin and his allies.

When a Designated Advocate Is Appropriate

When you first encounter a disability, you may have trouble coming to terms with the physical and emotional impact. You may not have the time, energy, motivation, or knowledge to advocate on your own behalf. If you feel this way, it is a good idea to have a designated advocate support you until you are able to take over your own case.

A designated advocate may assume some or all of the advocacy roles of people with degenerative conditions when the individual is no longer able to perform the necessary tasks. A designated advocate should be someone you trust, because he will make crucial decisions that will affect your life. Even if you are able to advocate on your own behalf, a friend, relative, or professional who has the time, expertise, and commitment to support your efforts can be helpful.

When a Citizen Advocate Is Appropriate

If you require a designated advocate but are unable to locate a family member or friend to work on your behalf, then a citizen advocate can be very helpful. Citizen advocates are usually volunteers who can be found through hospitals, physicians, social workers, paramedical personnel, and the clergy. Civic activists can also work as citizen advocates.

Case Study: Making Transit Accessible

In the early 1980s, the city of Hamilton, Ontario, had no transportation system for people with disabilities. People in the disability community had expressed their concerns to numerous politicians and other community leaders without success. Eventually, their cause reached a local community activist, who was angered by the absence of services to her constituents and decided to take action. On her own, she launched an effort to convince the city council to organize a transportation system that was accessible to people with mobility impairments and other disabilities. She wrote letters and made phone calls to convince city council members to set aside funding in the budget, and she solicited local automobile dealerships to donate or provide discounted vehicles that would make the system more effective. Bringing local businesses into her project offset the program's high start-up costs and ensured its success. Now people with disabilities in Hamilton have access to vans that pick them up at home, take them to their destination, and take them home again when they are finished. Hamilton has also purchased several accessible buses, further improving the transportation system.

When a Case Manager Is Appropriate

Case managers are most valuable when a disability first occurs, as they have the professional expertise to provide for all aspects of your care until you can do so on your own. Case managers can also offer valuable advice on how to fulfil advocacy roles and responsibilities. A case manager can even help guide you through a major advocacy initiative that you undertake on your own.

Renee

Renee was scheduled to undergo triple-bypass surgery. She had met with the surgeon who was scheduled to perform her operation, and found him very abrupt, cold, and impersonal. Although the surgeon was a qualified professional, his abrasive personality distressed her. Renee had a lot of anxiety about the operation, but when she asked her surgeon questions, he would give brusque answers. When she asked what the procedure entailed, his response was "You wouldn't understand. Don't worry about it." His answers made her more uneasy than ever. She shared her concerns with her case manager, Lois. When she realized the degree of her client's anxiety, Lois used her contacts within the local hospital system to arrange for another surgeon, one who was more communicative and empathetic, to perform the operation. On her own, Renee lacked the confidence and knowledge of the system that would have enabled her to change physicians.

When a Social Work–Sponsored Advocate Is Appropriate

It is appropriate to enlist the services of a social work–sponsored advocate when you are unable to handle the requirements of your care or of your advocacy efforts. These people play a role similar to that of a case manager, although they may not have the case manager's ability to intervene with medical professionals or to develop a complete program of care. They will often focus on your emotional well-being, and on locating and providing personnel for home and institutional care. One disadvantage to working with social work–sponsored advocates is that they often have a large caseload and may not always be able to devote sufficient time to your needs.

Roger

Roger worked as a fireman in Chicago. He was digging out a man who had become trapped when a sewer support structure collapsed, and he ruptured a disc in his back. As a result of this injury, he required extensive physiotherapy and chiropractic treatment. He was immobilized by his back problem, however, and could not attend regular clinics. Roger worked with a social worker, who arranged for a rotating series of volunteers from local universities and a local chiropractic college to come to his home to provide the necessary rehabilitation services. After six months of therapy, Roger had improved to the point where he could attend clinics on his own.

When Legal Advocates and Legal Clinics Are Appropriate

If individuals and organizations fail to respond to your requests after repeated notice, then legal action may be worthwhile. If your attorney does not specialize in or feel comfortable with disability issues, it may be worthwhile to approach a lawyer who specializes in this field. If you cannot afford to contract your own lawyer, legal clinics may be able to provide you with more reasonable support.

Ruth

Ruth had spina bifida, a congenital condition for which she often used a wheelchair. She worked as a media and product marketer, and moved to Toronto to pursue her career. At the first nine apartments Ruth saw, the landlords said that they were considering several applicants, and that they would let her know in the near future. Ruth was self-employed, had an established credit rating, was a non-smoker, and had three references. After being rejected by all nine landlords, she suspected that they were discriminating against her because of her disability. She contacted a lawyer, who wrote all nine landlords, stated that his client was financially secure, and suggested that their decisions appeared to be based on her disability, which was unacceptable and illegal. Within a week, Ruth was offered four of the apartments. The total cost for all of the lawyer's services was only fifty-seven dollars.

Ruth's story is not an isolated incident. Landlords have traditionally been very reluctant to rent their facilities to tenants with special needs. Lawyers have been successful in pressuring landlords not only to rent to clients with special needs, but also to renovate to accommodate their disabilities. Sometimes, a letter from a lawyer is all that is necessary, but on occasion, litigation is required. In almost all of these cases, legal advocacy is successful.

When a Special Advocate Is Appropriate

If you are advocating in a specific policy area (i.e., accommodation in educational or training programs, access issues, transportation requirements, government legislation, quality-of-life issues) and need information or guidance, a special advocate can be an invaluable resource. They can give you the advice you need or conduct a specific advocacy campaign on your behalf.

Ed

Ed was a lawyer in his mid-sixties who lost his eyesight after unsuccessful cataract surgery. A specialist who worked for the local institute for the blind assessed Ed's abilities and placed him in a training program where he learned Braille, adaptive walking skills, and living strategies so that he could cook, clean, and function at home and in the community. Ed embraced this program with great enthusiasm. His therapist was so impressed that she recruited him to become a special advocate working with people who had suddenly lost their sight. He now helps people who have gone blind learn to use computers, access social services, and design rehabilitation plans, and he instructs people on the use of seeing eye dogs, even though he himself chooses not to use one. Thanks to the help of a special advocate, Ed was able to become an advocate himself, and establish a new and productive career.

When Advocacy Groups Are Appropriate

Advocacy groups provide general expertise in all areas of advocacy, and can be particularly helpful if you are pursuing a change in legislation or a project that will have a broad impact on your community. Advocacy groups have numerous resources and will be able to provide you with a range of expertise that a single advocate may not be able to provide. If the advocacy group cannot provide the expertise or support you need, they will at least be able to put you in contact with someone who can.

Shaun

Shaun was a twenty-four-year-old man with cerebral palsy who had lived at home all his life. His parents were his primary caregivers, and they fed and clothed him. He enjoyed using swimming pools and other recreational facilities, and he spent a lot of time with friends, many of whom had significant disabilities. He felt socially isolated living with his parents, however, and wanted to move into an independent living centre (ILC), where he would be supported by caregivers but have more freedom to pursue his own schedule. His parents refused to allow him to leave. They told Shaun that he needed them, and then they accused him of being ungrateful for the lifelong care they had provided. Shaun, a counsellor from an ILC, and his friends approached a legal-advocacy clinic that provided services for people with disabilities. They intervened on Shaun's behalf, and convinced his parents to agree to a trial placement in the ILC. Shaun flourished in his new surroundings, where he enjoyed the full schedule of activities and was constantly surrounded by peers. This negotiated solution avoided what could have turned into a divisive court action between Shaun and his parents.

When Social Action Groups Are Appropriate
Social action groups are most helpful if you are trying to advocate for change on a state, provincial, or national level. Social action groups are plugged into key political networks, and have the resources to foster an effective lobbying campaign that may be beyond the capability of most disability groups.

Case Study: When Special-Interest Groups Work Together
Earlier we mentioned the impact of the Americans with Disabilities Act. This legislation was brought into being through the co-operation of disability groups and social action groups such as the National Association for the Advancement of Colored People (NAACP) and the American Civil Liberties Union (ACLU). These two groups had vast experience organizing national lobbying efforts. In the early 1980s, they began sharing information with leaders from disability groups on how to organize a successful lobby to initiate groundbreaking legislation. Once the

leaders in the disability lobby had "learned the ropes," the social action groups encouraged them to act on their own to increase their credibility. They eventually created an effective network whose power and legitimacy was recognized by George Bush, who adopted the ADA as part of his platform.

BECOMING A SUCCESSFUL ADVOCATE

The onset of disability almost always brings on a host of new needs. You may require specialized care, assistive computer technology, or custom-designed equipment, or you may have to overcome discrimination. If you take control of your situation, educate yourself about your disability, and prepare yourself thoroughly for each advocacy effort you undertake, you stand an excellent chance of success.

Take Control

Taking control means asserting power over your own life and ensuring that no one but you or your designated advocate makes your most important decisions. You can retain control of your life following disability by making your wishes known to others and engaging the appropriate legal protection. In the event that you are unable to communicate effectively, legal tools such as the power of attorney (see Chapter 13) can ensure that decisions are made in accordance with your wishes.

Educate Yourself

Before you can make concrete decisions, you need information. Becoming fully informed about your disability is one of the most important steps you can take to ensure that your efforts are worthwhile. Not everyone is aware of his own needs, or of how these needs can be met. Only after you have become informed about your disability will you be able to determine the best approach.

Education will familiarize you with the people, resources, and services that are available to help you reach your goals.

You can gather information from local libraries, physicians, and support groups. Newsletters, magazines, and conferences held by disability associations can also keep you up to date on the most important advances and techniques. One of the best sources of information on disability, and the one that is expanding most rapidly, is the Internet, which is discussed later in this book.

Prepare Yourself

You will always find it easier to gain accommodation for your needs if you are well prepared. Prior to launching any advocacy effort, you should try to determine exactly what you want, why you are entitled to it, and how it can be implemented. Consulting support groups, legal clinics, or lawyers can be particularly helpful. They should be able to provide you with accurate information on any technical matters, as well as direct you to other useful resources.

Don't Reinvent the Wheel

Always remember to try the easy route first. A program you need may already exist — it might just be hard to find. Someone in your community may be able to provide what you need, or put you in touch with an individual or organization that can help you out. Asking the right person or group for help may provide a quick solution to your problem, and save you a lot of trouble and aggravation. Local support groups usually have the resources to meet most of your needs. Move on to more complex strategies only after you have established that what you need is not currently available.

If the program or item you are looking for does not exist, it may be because no one has ever expressed a need for it before. If this is the case, all you may have to do is make a request to the proper authorities.

THE ART OF PERSUASION

When you have laid the groundwork for your advocacy efforts by learning about your condition and preparing your case, the next step is to approach the people and organizations that have the influence or the power to grant your request. The following techniques will help make your advocacy efforts more effective.

State Your Case Clearly

A reluctance or refusal to accommodate people with disabilities often stems from ignorance or lack of sensitivity, rather than malice. If you can show that your needs are legitimate, that you have the support of the law, and that you have a reasonable solution to the problem, you should have a better chance for success.

Be Organized

If you prepare all relevant information in a coherent fashion, it will make your case more compelling. If you are disorganized, the group with whom you are negotiating will be more likely to ignore your concerns. Thorough documentation that supports the legitimacy of your request is an important part of a comprehensive presentation. Sharing examples of similar accommodations made in other jurisdictions and demonstrating the legitimacy of these measures can help you avoid a protracted struggle.

Focus on Problem-Solving

Always keep in mind that your ultimate goal is to get your needs met, not to embarrass or punish your adversary. Try to avoid confrontation, as most people will be more resistant to your requests if they feel intimidated or threatened. If they continue to be unresponsive, however, you may have to use more aggressive techniques.

Recruit Allies

If you are advocating on an issue that affects a wide range of people, enlist allies to support your efforts. Decision-makers will be more receptive if you can convince them that the accommodations you seek will improve the lives of a significant number of other people as well. Your allies' knowledge and expertise can supplement your abilities, and they can also provide moral, emotional, financial, and legal support.

WHAT IF MY INITIAL APPROACH IS UNSUCCESSFUL?

Although it is best to try to reach a negotiated solution, a forceful, well-reasoned presentation may not be enough to sway intransigent people or organizations. If your legitimate request is refused, don't give up; you just have to try another tack.

Return to Your Support Group

The odds are that someone in your support group has undergone a similar experience. They will be able to share both the strategies that worked and the ones that didn't work for them, and suggest alternative strategies for you to use.

Try a Public Education Campaign

Media exposure can alert entire communities to your cause, providing you with added support and putting pressure on the relevant parties to take action. You can begin the campaign by sending letters, faxes, or e-mails to the individual or organization that has been unresponsive, and sending copies to important people, key organizations, and the media to gain attention and mobilize support for your demands. These letters should restate both your goals and the steps you have taken to have them addressed, as well as the circumstances surrounding your adversary's refusal. Give your counterpart the opportunity to respond to public pressure before pursuing legal action.

Use Politicians

The name of the game is power. Sometimes public pressure is not enough, and you have to appeal to those members of your community who have the power to effect change. Politicians can often be convinced to amend a wide range of laws to make them disability-friendly, and they may be able to convince landlords to abide by existing regulations.

Local politicians and community leaders are elected to serve their constituents, and they are almost always willing to accommodate people with special needs who have a legitimate grievance. They do so for two reasons: first, to uphold the law; and second, to remain popular with the electorate. When you discuss disability issues with politicians, be aware of both of these interests.

Consider Legal Action

Usually, the effective use of media and political pressure will allow you to achieve your goals without having to rely on the court system. If these further public advocacy efforts are unsuccessful, however, you should consult a lawyer or legal clinic that specializes in disability-related law. It may also be advisable to contact a local university law faculty or a legal clinic. The faculty or clinic can offer strategies to help you obtain your requests on a *pro bono* basis.

WHAT IF I LIVE IN A SMALL COMMUNITY?

In small communities, the personnel, technology, and programs you need may not always be available. In some cases, relocating to a larger community may provide the access you're seeking. In other cases, such as when the technology you need is new or unavailable, a local engineer or carpenter may be able to build it for you. Local service clubs and church organizations can also help with your advocacy efforts.

Case Study: Making a Big Difference in a Small Town

Mount Pleasant is a small farming town in Ontario. It did not have any specialized facilities for seniors with disabilities, although there were many retired farmers in the surrounding area who could have benefited from such a service. The mayor of the town and a local minister, together with two children who were concerned about their parents' ability to continue living on their own, recognized the need for a community living centre for local senior citizens with disabilities. This would mean that retired farmers could move into an accessible caregiving facility without having to move to a big city.

This group of four began to raise the issue at town council meetings, service club meetings, and at their local churches. Within a couple of weeks, they had attracted fifty people who were willing to volunteer time and effort. The group then lobbied bank managers, local businessmen, church leaders, service club representatives, and local government officials to help them build the facility. They raised enough money to buy a pre-existing apartment building, which they had rezoned for group living and retrofitted for people with disabilities. They undertook an extensive renovation to instal kitchen and washroom facilities, a social hall, and a gymnasium. After the building was completed, they hired full-time staff to manage the facility, which accommodated twenty-nine retirees from the community. By taking action and rallying people to their cause, these four people were able to make a big difference in their community.

CONCLUSION

Advocacy is a valuable skill that you can use in all areas of your life. It will provide you with organizational skills, a clear focus, and the confidence to ensure the best possible care and treatment. Advocacy can also ensure access to opportunities in all aspects of your life. With hard work, the advocacy attitude, and a little patience and training, you can obtain the best results. When other people realize that you are knowledgeable and committed, they are more likely to work with you to solve your problems.

Chapter

6

The Law Is on
Your Side!

INTRODUCTION

The law can be a powerful weapon for people with disabilities. Not only are all people legally protected from discrimination on the basis of disability, but governments and private businesses must take "positive steps" to ensure that people with disabilities can gain access to and benefit from everything that is available to the general public. Governments and businesses must take action to remove barriers that exclude or encumber people with disabilities, and they cannot discriminate against people with special needs in their employment policies.

If you encounter resistance in your advocacy work, do not be afraid to ask for or demand what you need and, if necessary, go to court. This chapter will explain your rights, how to obtain those rights without a lawyer, when to engage the services of a lawyer, and how to pursue legal action. In Chapter 13, the section on legal planning explains the measures you can take to ensure that you and your family are protected in the event of partial or total disability.

PROTECTION UNDER THE LAW

The Americans with Disabilities Act in the United States and the Charter of Rights and Freedoms in Canada both guarantee the rights of people with disabilities. The ADA prohibits discrimination on the basis of disability in employment, programs, and services provided by state and local governments; in services provided by private companies; and in commercial facilities. Section 15 of the Canadian Charter of Rights and Freedoms provides general protection in a wide range of fields.

The intent of the law in both countries is to promote the integration of people with disabilities by requiring that all reasonable steps be taken to ensure equal treatment. The ADA separates society's responsibility to people with disabilities into five categories: employment, public services, public accommodations, telecommunications, and miscellaneous. In Canada, the protections are not as explicitly defined, but they have usually been enforced whenever a legal challenge has been mounted.

Employment

Employers must make "reasonable accommodation" to protect the rights of individuals with disabilities in all aspects of their employment. Examples of "reasonable accommodation" include restructuring a job, making existing facilities readily accessible to and usable by employees with disabilities, modifying work schedules, altering the layout of workstations, reassigning a current employee to a more suitable vacant position for which the individual is qualified, and acquiring or modifying equipment. Discrimination is prohibited in hiring and firing, the application process, the awarding of wages and benefits

120

(including health insurance), leave, and all other employment-related activities.

Public Services

Public services — which include all national, state, provincial, and local government institutions; national rail and air travel corporations; and commuter authorities — cannot deny services to people with disabilities. Any programs or activities that are open to people without disabilities must also be accessible to individuals with disabilities. These include public-transportation systems such as buses and subways. For example, since 1990, all buses that have been manufactured in the U.S. for public transit have been wheelchair-accessible. Airlines have made similar accommodations for people with special needs, such as providing wider aisles and mobility aids.

Public Accommodations

All new public buildings and renovated existing buildings must be accessible to people with disabilities. Barriers to services in existing facilities must be removed if this is readily achievable. Public accommodations include restaurants, hotels, grocery stores, and retail stores, as well as privately owned transportation systems. Wheelchair ramps are now a standard component of any building plan, and most public washrooms have been retrofitted with grab bars and other devices to make them easier for people with disabilities to use.

Telecommunications

Companies offering telecommunications to the general public must make telephone-relay service available to individuals who use devices for hearing and sight impairments. People who are unable to dial can speak numbers into a phone, which will then be automatically dialed. Service providers are mandated by law to make this feature available.

Miscellaneous

The law prohibits coercing, threatening, or retaliating against people with disabilities or those who attempt to aid people with disabilities in asserting their rights. For example, it used to be a common practice to eject tenants from rental accommodations after they experienced a physical or mental disability. It is now almost impossible for a landlord to evict or discriminate against tenants on the basis of disability.

WHAT IS "REASONABLE"?

The legislation protecting the rights of people with disabilities hinges on the words "reasonable accommodation." An employer or business will not be required to make an accommodation if it can be demonstrated that the changes would impose "undue hardship" on the operation of the business. An undue hardship is an action that causes a business "significant difficulty or expense" in relation to its size, the resources available, and the nature of the operation. Undue hardship must be determined on a case-by-case basis. For example, building a ramp and making washrooms accessible would not constitute an undue hardship.

COMMON LEGAL PROBLEMS

Even though the law is on your side, sometimes people and companies will resist meeting their legal obligations. There are several common problem areas.

Resistance to Accommodation

Businesses and other organizations will often be reluctant to accede to your wishes. This is to be expected, as most organizations do not want to spend more money than they absolutely have to. Do not be intimidated if someone suggests that the accommodations you seek constitute an "undue hardship." It is always worthwhile to investigate the real costs and consequences of providing special accommodations — don't just take someone's word for it.

Until recently, taxi cabs, airplanes, trains, and buses refused to allow people with visual impairments, who were accompanied by guide dogs, to use their services. This made travelling very difficult. In the early 1990s, people with visual and hearing impairments launched a series of lawsuits aimed at increasing accessibility to public transportation. These cases were all successful, and as a result, guide dogs are now permitted on all forms of public transportation.

Resistance to Entering and Re-entering the Workplace

The law requires that people who return to their jobs after suffering a disability be given the opportunity to resume their responsibilities. Many organizations, however, will hesitate or even refuse to reinstate workers with disabilities to their previous positions or to positions that offer similar responsibilities and compensation. If they fail to reinstate you, refuse to make the changes necessary to accommodate you, put undue pressure on you, or do not give you an adequate opportunity to resume your position, you may be required to engage legal counsel.

People cannot be fired because they have a disability, but they can be fired if they are unable to perform their duties. As a result, individuals who return to the workplace after sustaining a permanent disability often find themselves under increased pressure, and are sometimes judged by harsher standards than other employees. There is a flawed perception in society that people with significant disabilities can't perform as well as people without disabilities. Because of this, some employers look for an excuse to terminate an employee with a disability.

Gina

Gina worked as a secretary for an executive in a large investment firm. She lived in Baltimore, and was married with two children. In a two-week period one December, both of her elderly parents passed away. Gina had always been close to her mother and father, and their deaths triggered a severe bout of depression. She took four weeks off work to receive psychotherapy to help her cope with her losses. When she returned, her boss told her that she had been fired and was being offered six months' severance pay. In spite of her eleven years of good service, Gina was terminated because her boss did not want to employ someone with "psychiatric problems." Gina retained an attorney, who wrote to the company outlining Gina's legitimate grievance and threatened legal action if she was not reinstated with compensation. The lawyer made the company aware of the strength of Gina's case, and within three days she was reinstated.

LEGAL SOLUTIONS TO PROBLEMS

In the previous chapter, we discussed addressing the problems you may encounter through advocacy. Although the vast majority of problems can be resolved through non-legal means, it may be appropriate to pursue legal action if you have exhausted all of your alternatives.

Different Types of Legal Initiatives

Although the details of each case are different, the legal actions pursued by people with disabilities can be grouped into several broad categories.

A. Gaining the Enforcement of Established Provisions. Sometimes rights and entitlements are firmly established, but a group or organization may refuse to provide them. In such a scenario, a lawsuit or the threat of legal action may be necessary. These legal actions have forced landlords to make buildings accessible, and employers to make workplaces barrier-free and free of contaminants that can cause disability. The law has also been used to force accommodations in the workplace.

Case Study: Curing a Sick Building

A group of office workers who shared the same building in Toledo began to suffer from nausea, headaches, respiratory problems, and eye irritation at a very high rate. They worked in a building that was built in the early 1960s, and they suspected that the cause of their ailments was environmental. The owner held that there was nothing wrong with the building, but after numerous tenant complaints, building and health officials were invited to inspect the premises. Their investigations revealed that the building contained large amounts of asbestos, some of which was being circulated through the ventilation system. The building was found to be in contravention of local health and safety legislation, but the landlord was reluctant to comply with the necessary renovations, which would have been expensive. The inspectors took the landlord to court, where he was directed by the judge to remove all asbestos from the building. After the asbestos was removed, the workers' health returned to normal. The law will almost always protect you from having to work in unsafe conditions.

B. Restitution for Negligence. If an individual or organization causes a disability through negligence or malpractice, they can be held criminally, civilly, and financially liable. These liabilities may include covering of the costs of disability and punitive damages, and may even result in imprisonment or fines.

Corey

Corey suffered from a blockage of his arteries, and he was scheduled to undergo corrective bypass surgery. In the course of his operation, however, the surgeon accidentally cut open his aortic valve, leading to massive blood loss. Although the average human has only nine pints of blood in his system, Corey required the transfusion of twenty pints of blood during his surgery to keep him alive. After the surgery, it became apparent that he had moderate brain damage. He was also in a permanent state of physical weakness, and he had to give up his profession. Corey and his family sued the doctors and the hospital for malpractice, and they won a multi-million dollar settlement. This did not make up for the loss of his occupation and the diminution of his quality of life, but it eased the long-term financial burden of Corey's care.

C. Establishing New Legal Precedents. People with disabilities and their advocates will sometimes mount legal challenges in order to gain new rights or compensation for themselves and other people with disabilities. Precedents may involve the establishment of a new law, winning a new interpretation of an old law to address the needs of people with disabilities, or getting controversial conditions defined as disabilities (these have included carpal tunnel syndrome, post-traumatic stress syndrome, and burnout).

My Story

Because I am unable to write, I require the assistance of a secretary for all of my university-related course work, academic research, and correspondence. Secretarial fees usually cost me between $10,000 and $15,000 a year. Without the help of a secretary, it would be impossible for me to fulfil my duties. In my first year as a professor, I claimed my secretarial expenses as a business deduction, in exactly the same way as a business would deduct the cost of purchasing computers or any other necessary equipment. My claim was denied when Revenue Canada ruled that an employee could not have another employee do his or her work. I launched a legal battle that went to the Supreme Court of Canada and was ultimately decided in my favour.

Unfortunately, as a direct result of my case, the tax department revised the tax code, giving a credit of approximately $1,500 to all people who submit medical proof that they have a disability. In some years, I use up this tax credit in one month. It is not sufficient to cover my disability-related work costs. This cap on work-related expenses hinders many people with disabilities. Almost all Western countries, except for Canada, allow these deductions.

D. Lawsuits Stemming from Perceptions of Prejudice and Discrimination. When people with disabilities are treated unfairly, or are prevented from earning an income by discriminatory policies, they often have little recourse but to go to court. These lawsuits are used to gain access to educational and recreational programs, and to challenge discriminatory hiring and employment practices.

Casey Martin

Casey Martin is an accomplished young golfer who is attempting to launch a career on the Professional Golfers' Association (PGA) tour. Martin is affected by Klippel-Trenaunay-Weber syndrome, a congenital circulatory disorder in his lower right leg that makes it impossible for him to play an eighteen-hole golf course without the use of a cart. However, the PGA is adamantly opposed to allowing any players to ride a cart during tournaments. Using the Americans with Disabilities Act, Martin gained an injunction against the PGA tour's rule. Once Martin was allowed to compete, he met with success, winning the first tournament he entered and finishing in the top twenty-five at the 1998 U.S. Open. Without the ADA, it is unlikely that Martin would have been allowed to compete, but, given the opportunity, he clearly demonstrated that he is able to golf at a professional level.

Casey Martin has drawn support from numerous sources, including Bob Dole and Tiger Woods, who said, "I think it would be great for the tour. It's like seeing Jim Abbott [a pitcher with only one hand who played major league baseball] out there pitching. . . . He was such a hero, with one hand, doing the things he was able to do. I looked up to him." Martin would clearly be a role model for all people with disabilities, and it would be very unfortunate if this discriminatory policy was allowed to stand. His first court action was decided in his favour, and he was allowed to use a cart on the Nike tour and in several PGA tournaments.

HOW TO TAKE EFFECTIVE LEGAL ACTION

The first thing to do if you are considering legal action is to find effective representation. You can consider a lawyer, legal clinic, paralegal, or university law school. Many lawyers specialize in disability-related law and have great expertise in the area. Finding someone with a good reputation is especially important in the legal field. In many jurisdictions, lawyer referral services will provide recommendations of qualified professionals.

Once you have launched legal action, your lawyer will be

responsible for the technical details of your case. Discuss your case with her on an ongoing basis so you remain fully informed. Be honest and open with your lawyer, and explicitly set out your objectives — why you are pursuing the case and what you hope to achieve. It is usually a good idea to listen to your legal representative. Your lawyer can tell you what you may be entitled to, where the law stands on your issue, and the range of possible outcomes. If you stay informed and have a good working relationship, you should be well served by your attorney.

Settlement vs. Trial

In many disability-related disputes, the defendant sometimes offers a settlement to avoid the substantial costs of trial. If the settlement meets all of your needs, then it is usually wise to accept it. However, most defendants will be unwilling to provide full compensation. Have in mind an amount that you are willing to settle for, and that will meet all your needs. If the offer does not meet your bottom line, consider pursuing the case further. Financial settlements are discussed in more detail in the chapter on disability planning.

If you are trying to set a precedent, a settlement that refuses to recognize in law the rights you are pursuing will generally be insufficient. If you are committed to achieving systemic change, you may be forced to go all the way. As a precedent-setting court case requires great sacrifice, it is a good idea to enlist allies to help develop your case and to defray the costs. Advocacy groups, support groups, and social-action groups are the best sources of this support.

CONCLUSION

We have achieved rapid and significant change through the legal system. By aggressively pushing for constitutional rights and accommodations, people with disabilities have gained more freedom, independence, and access to the workplace. But there is still a lot of work to be done. Many buildings are not fully accessible, and people with disabilities still routinely experience discrimination. Legislative protection means that if this happens to you, you have recourse. The name of the game is power. If you have the backing of advocacy and support groups, you will be able to obtain the protection and benefits to which you are entitled.

PART 2

Caring for People with Disabilities

Chapter 7

Caregiving for People with Disabilities

INTRODUCTION

I would never have been able to make it without the help of my caregivers. When I was growing up, my parents, siblings, cousins, aunts, uncles, and friends spent hours helping me exercise, learn to ride a bike, and look after myself. I even remember them teaching me how to walk, because I did not learn until I was five years old. They were patient and encouraging, and they taught me never to give up. My parents and fellow classmates also helped me through school, by taking notes and writing out assignments from my dictation.

My caregivers were just as important after my heart attacks. My wife, Sharon, and son David visited me every day in the hospital, my son Adam came home from school to visit me on weekends, and many of my friends came to provide company and support, and to bring me food that wasn't from the hospital cafeteria. If you are constantly surrounded by friends and family, it is easier to maintain a positive outlook and to keep up the strength that you need to recover. Caregivers can make all the difference.

Caregiving isn't always easy. If you assume responsibility for the care of a loved one, you will have to work hard, learn new skills, and manage stress. Caregiving is more than just an aggregation of different physical tasks. In addition to performing all of the physical requirements of care, you also have to look after your own health and home, and manage and plan long-term care. If you are organized, prepared, and committed, you will be able to do all of these things and make a tremendous and positive difference. This chapter provides ideas and suggestions that can help you negotiate the challenges of disability.

A CAREGIVER'S RESPONSIBILITIES

If someone you love experiences a disability, it is your responsibility as the primary caregiver to take control of the situation. There are a number of important questions you have to ask:

- Is our home still the best place for us to live?
- If so, do we need to make any changes?
- Will we need to bring in any personnel?
- What new tasks will I now have to take responsibility for?
- Who is there to help and support me? (Perhaps the most important question of all.)

If you are the primary caregiver for your spouse or partner, you may be responsible for a range of tasks that go beyond physical caregiving. These include managing changing roles within your family; maintaining your children's discipline and shared involvement in caregiving; arranging transportation; scheduling medical and rehabilitative appointments; arranging for recreation; helping with rehabilitation exercises; and most important, providing your partner with personal support, encouragement, and love. Work with your spouse to achieve the maximum possible level of freedom, and encourage him to do everything that he can on his own.

Maintaining your duties over an extended period of time can be more difficult than adjusting to the initial responsibilities of providing care. When disability first occurs, a burst of adrenaline can make it easier to maintain a high level of energy and rise to the occasion. For the first while, you may be able to arrange or provide a high-level of care while "keeping your head above water" both at work and at home. This manic pace cannot be maintained forever. Performing multiple roles over months and even years can be exceptionally draining. **Don't try to do everything alone!**

Thomas

Thomas was a sixty-two-year-old executive with a mining company. He had been married to his wife, Beatrice, for almost forty years, and they had three grown children. Thomas collapsed at work one day and was taken to the emergency ward, where he was diagnosed as having had a stroke. He experienced severe weakness on his left side, and his right leg was paralysed. He began to stutter as well. Thomas could not walk without assistance, and at first he could not feed himself or hold a glass or a cup. He also required assistance when going to the bathroom and bathing. After he'd spent three weeks in the hospital, Beatrice decided that she would be able to provide the necessary care at home.

For the first week, Beatrice was able to care for Thomas without too much difficulty. Although she was tired at the end of the week, both were satisfied with the arrangement. She was the sole caregiver and was responsible for her husband twenty-four hours a day, seven days a week, even though her children visited often to provide meals, company, and moral support. With each successive day, Beatrice found the requirements of care to be more and more difficult. By the end of the third week, she had had enough. The physical strain of constantly supporting Thomas and maintaining a hectic twenty-four-hour schedule was more than she could handle at fifty-nine.

Beatrice wanted to continue as sole caregiver, but her children and family physician had noticed that she was reaching the point of exhaustion, and they intervened. They counselled her to hire two caregivers on a part-time basis and to use community supports. She agreed. Although she remained in charge of caregiving, Beatrice no longer had to perform most of the physical tasks of care. She was able to regain her strength, concentrate on motivating her husband to rehabilitate, and reinforce the bonds of their relationship.

Many people will be ready and willing to provide support, and some will volunteer their services. Others may be reluctant to become involved, however, as they may fear intruding in your private life or feel that they do not have the skills to help. Ask for support when you need it. People will be there to help.

Contact support personnel early, even before you return home and settle into a caregiving routine, if possible. Support specialists can answer any questions you may have, and will help to design a program and schedule for care. If you contact them after you have initiated a care program, they can encourage you to continue with the things you are doing right and let you know what you can change or improve. Support staff can also provide contacts, information, and services that will make your job easier.

Disability in the Family

I recently spoke to a woman whose husband had just had a stroke and was unable to leave his bed or communicate effectively. "I don't even know how to talk to my husband any more. What do I say and what do I do?" My response was: "Try to treat him as you always have: with warmth, with dignity, with respect, and with love."

If a loved one experiences a disability, don't talk down to him, ignore him, or treat him like a child. Many people who have lost their ability to communicate still understand everything. Being treated as an adult is a strong motivator for those who have the capacity to improve. If someone has difficulty communicating or comprehending conversation, or if you must wait a longer time for a response, resist the inclination to simplify everything and talk to him as if he is a child. Mental stimulation is essential to rehabilitation.

As the main caregiver and decision-maker, you are trying to provide as much independence and stimulation as possible. Include the recipient of care in decision-making, and bring in friends and family members as frequently as possible. Music often has a soothing effect, and can help in rehabilitation. Radio and television can also be effective sources of stimulation, but you should not use television as the substitute for a proper rehabilitation program or human contact. If the patient can use the Internet, a home hook-up is an excellent conduit to the outside world. It provides people to talk to, is a constant source of the most up-to-date information on medical conditions, and offers anything else one might find of interest.

Learning New Tasks and Skills

If your partner experiences a serious disability that temporarily or permanently limits his motor skills, you may have to help him with bathing, toileting, eating, personal grooming, medicating, getting in and out of bed, getting dressed, and many other tasks that you likely never expected to perform.

These tasks can be very stressful if repeated on a regular basis, but a skilled therapist can show you the easiest way to perform each of them. Nonetheless, you may want to bring in outside caregivers to assist you. Outside caregivers can be family members, friends, volunteers, or paid professionals.

Disability may also require you to learn some new skills that are not directly related to the condition, as you may be called on to assume some of your partner's roles on a temporary or permanent basis. These may include accounting, paying the bills, investing, cooking, shopping, taking care of the children, repairing your home and car, and cleaning. These are all in addition to your regular responsibilities. One person cannot do the work of two for an extended period of time. To prevent becoming overburdened, you have to organize your responsibilities, share your tasks as broadly as possible, and maintain time to "recharge your batteries."

COPING WITH THE STRESS OF CAREGIVING

Caregiving can be draining, and family members who expend all of their energy providing care are at risk of burnout. Rest, relaxation, and recreation are absolute necessities. Everyone has to maintain his own space. Respite care and outside support are excellent means of providing a break, and in the long run will increase the quality of care you can provide.

In Chapter 2, we discussed some of the signs of negative coping with disability. These included anger, avoidance, and taking away independence. As a caregiver, you must guard against engaging in any of these behaviours. If you notice that you are exhibiting some of the signs of negative coping, you must enlist added support to provide respite care or to ease your caregiving schedule. Counselling may also be helpful.

Know when you have reached your limits. Don't try to be Supercaregiver, the hero who can do anything and everything. Bringing in other caregivers on a temporary or permanent basis is not an acknowledgment of failure, but part of an essential strategy to provide your loved one with the best possible care. In addition to easing the stress of caregiving, outsiders can add a new perspective to care. They often see things differently, and may be able to suggest new strategies that did not occur to you.

Brian

Brian was thirty-two when he was in a serious car accident. He had neck injuries, a shoulder separation, a broken knee, and many cuts and bruises. He received 437 stitches and had to recuperate in the hospital for two weeks. When he returned home, he was very angry at being in pain and at facing the prospect of not being able to return to work as an electrician immediately. He was frustrated and embarrassed by the fact that he was forced to rely on his wife and children during the initial stages of his recovery. His wife and children tried to be supportive, but they were unable to cheer him up and he started yelling at them on a regular basis.

His wife, Sarah, went to their family doctor, who recommended that they bring in an outside caregiver. The new caregiver was a forty-two-year-old professional caregiver named Peter, who had fifteen years' experience working with sick and injured patients. The first time Brian took out his anger on Peter, Peter took exception and read Brian the riot act. He threatened to quit on the spot if Brian ever again swore or used an aggressive tone of voice with him or any members of the family. This was a turning-point in Brian's rehabilitation. He realized that his behaviour had been inappropriate, and he began to control his emotional outbursts. Peter continued to work with the family for five months, and nine months later Brian was able to return to work.

If possible, select a caregiver jointly with your spouse and other family members. The criteria that are most important are skills, reliability, commitment, a personal rapport with the recipient of the care, and a willingness to listen.

Respite Care

Everyone involved in caring for someone with special needs will require periods of rest and relaxation. Respite care, in which volunteers or professionals temporarily replace regular caregivers, is one of the best ways to provide these breaks. Respite care allows regular caregivers to take a vacation, unwind, or even learn new caregiving techniques from support groups, professionals, or conferences. Caregivers will return from these breaks refreshed and able to continue providing quality care. Respite care can be provided by other family members, professional caregivers, or volunteers, and can take place in your home or in an institutional setting. Many seniors' residences and nursing homes have extra rooms and staff available to provide respite care for seniors with disabilities.

Respite caregivers may not always provide the same quality of care as family members and permanent professional caregivers. Although respite caregivers may not have the same level of commitment or skills as regular caregivers, most of them, if properly trained and supervised, will be able to serve your purposes. Some people with disabilities come to feel dependent on their primary caregiver, and they may react negatively to the efforts of replacements. If you are careful when selecting and evaluating personnel, problems with respite care can be avoided.

THE IMPORTANCE OF A SUPPORT NETWORK

Disability can put stress on your working life, your family life, and your social life. Don't try to handle it all on your own. Disability can make people feel that they are isolated and alone, but nothing could be further from the truth. There are many individuals who are willing and able to assist you, and there are thousands of organizations across the continent that are specially designed to provide support for people with disabilities. Support networks can provide you with the answers to many of your questions, and save you a lot of time, effort, and heartache.

WHAT IS A SUPPORT NETWORK?

A support network is composed of all of the individuals and groups who provide the assistance, advice, and support that you need to cope with your disability. First and foremost, the network is composed of the family and friends who are committed to your care. They will be your most steadfast source of support, the ones you can count on at any time of the day or night. A network may also include the local or national chapter of a support group for your disability, advocacy groups, caregivers, medical or paramedical personnel, religious groups, and community service clubs. By using all of these resources, you can ensure that you will not have to face your disability alone.

Taking advantage of the services offered by existing support groups will help to guarantee that the support you require will always be available. Accessing community groups is another necessary step in developing the resources to help you cope. A successful support network can ease the burden on caregivers, provide creative solutions to problems, and make you secure in the knowledge that your needs will be looked after. Over an extended period of time, support networks are essential in preventing burnout and helping maintain a high level of care.

THE COMPONENTS OF A SUPPORT NETWORK

Family and Friends

Although they may not initially have experience or expertise in dealing with a disability, close family members and friends are important sources of support for many people. Family and friends provide caring social, emotional, and physical support, and they can almost always be relied upon in emergencies. Friends and family members who can take your mind off your disability over lunch, a movie, or a simple visit can be just as important as any doctor or therapist. After you encounter a disability, your life does not stop. Maintaining social contact is crucial to your self-esteem and your ability to get on with life.

The support of family and friends is equally important to your spouse or partner. Providing care for a person with a disability, especially a loved one, can be emotionally and physically draining. After I had my heart attacks and surgery, my friend Jack would come by and say, "Mark, let's go." He would make me get up, no matter how tired I was, and we would go for lunch or a drive. Although I did not have much energy in the months following my surgery, a change of scenery was absolutely essential for my well-being. Equally important were the times when our friends Sandy, Sondrea, and Lynne would come by to take my wife, Sharon, out to lunch. They would tell me, "Mark, we love you, but you are not invited." They realized that as my principal caregiver, Sharon needed time out from caring for me so she could avoid the problems associated with burnout. Support networks are as important for caregivers as they are for those who have disabilities.

Support Groups

Support groups are made up of individuals who have experienced a particular disability and their supporters. The members are familiar with the best strategies for solving problems associated with specific conditions. Support groups provide current information on your condition, as well as the entire range of personnel and therapies available for your treatment. They offer advice on medical professionals, treatment facilities, and the latest technologies, and they may even provide equipment at little or no charge. Perhaps most important, support groups provide an atmosphere in which you can feel comfortable, since you're surrounded by people who have had similar experiences and who understand what you are going through. Because of this shared experience, members of support groups can offer advice and solutions that may not occur to professionals and others who have not experienced a disability.

Support groups are usually organized at the national, state or provincial, and local levels, and include organizations such as the Heart and Stroke Foundation and the national institutes for the blind and the hearing impaired. They can be located in most large urban communities, and they exist for almost every form of disability. If there is no local chapter in your region, you can contact the organization through its national, state, or provincial office, or through your community's social service information network. A directory of some of these organizations appears in Appendix B. Support groups are there for everyone who needs them, and they look to recruit new members all the time. They welcome anyone who is affected by a disability, including the family members of people with special needs.

Disability Organizations (Local)

Local chapters of support groups will provide you with a wealth of information, resources, and understanding. In an environment of people who have shared similar experiences, you can vent your frustrations, fears, and hopes, and work together with group members to identify and fulfil mutual needs. Fellow members can offer information about the medical personnel, treatments, and resources in your community. They can also help you evaluate therapies and raise funds for group and individual programs.

Disability-specific organizations sometimes provide equipment such as wheelchairs, prosthetics, and computers at reasonable prices. If they do not have these devices on hand, they will be able to direct you to the most reliable suppliers. In some cases, members can construct specialized equipment at substantially lower rates than what are commercially available. Perhaps most important, these groups provide education for individuals, their family members, their caregivers, and the general public.

Disability Organizations (National and International)

Larger budgets and higher levels of membership enable parent organizations to advocate for their causes on a national and international level, as well as engage in large-scale corporate and personal fund-raising to support research and provide resources for member groups and individuals. Disability-specific groups at the national level often serve as co-ordinators and fund-raisers for their local chapters. The Muscular Dystrophy Association of America is one well-known example. Because of its high profile, which has developed through the Jerry Lewis Telethon and other charitable activities, it has raised hundreds of millions of dollars and increased national awareness and sensitivity to muscular dystrophy. The funds that have been raised by this group and others, such as the American Cancer Society, have been put towards research that may one day result in a cure.

This research would not be possible without the co-ordinating abilities of the national offices, which provide equally valuable information services. National foundations are in constant contact with medical researchers who keep them abreast of the latest innovations, which they then share with their member organizations. New techniques and innovations are passed from the national to the local chapters, which do not have the same access to the research.

Service Clubs
Service clubs are local, national, or international organizations whose main objective is to improve the quality of life of the citizens in their communities. Even though some of them represent specific ethnic, cultural, or religious groups, they usually offer a broad range of services to all members of the community. Service clubs can provide financial assistance and equipment that will make your life easier. The Shriners, the Elks, the Kinsmen, Kiwanis, the Rotary, B'nai Brith, and many other groups provide services to people with disabilities. Many service groups have contributed funds to finding donors for people who require bone-marrow transplants and offsetting the costs of surgery. Service groups provided the essential support that enabled the creation of international registries of bone-marrow donors, which have saved thousands of lives.

Phil, a retired insurance salesman who had been widowed for five years, lived in a seniors' residence in downtown Toronto. He had a great deal of difficulty moving around, owing to a severe back injury that caused him to use a wheelchair part of the time. He was a former member of the local Kiwanis Club, and a fellow member heard of his difficulties. He arranged for the local chapter of the club to use some of the funds it had raised in a charity banquet to redesign Phil's apartment to make it accessible. All of the passageways were widened, and his counters and sinks were lowered. These renovations enabled Phil to remain independent.

Religious Organizations

Religious organizations serve a purpose similar to service clubs, but they usually focus their efforts on members of their own congregations. They provide personal services, such as counselling, visitation, and hospital care, and will occasionally offer financial support. Religious faith can also help people to come to terms with their disability. Rabbis, ministers, priests, and other religious leaders are often expert counsellors, and they will provide essential emotional support for all members of families affected by disability.

Nick was a thirty-one-year-old father of three who lived in Fairmount, California. He sustained multiple injuries after falling from a ladder. His back and right knee were severely damaged, and he was unable to work. Nick was self-employed, and had not purchased sufficient health and disability insurance. As a result, he did not receive the medical care and therapy that were required. He was good friends with his minister, who was aware of Nick's difficulties. The minister, from a local Anglican diocese, asked a physiotherapist and chiropractor to provide assessments and therapy on a voluntary basis. These services were delivered free of charge for more than two years, and they were instrumental in helping Nick return to work.

Some religious groups have a more organized and institutional approach to disability, which frequently takes the form of a volunteer committee that arranges to have services provided for members in need. Some church groups even help congregants protect themselves from the impact of disability by organizing discounted rates for disability- and life-insurance policies for their members.

Community Volunteers

Community volunteers are essential for people who do not have a network of family or professional support. Community volunteers can fill most of the roles of a primary family caregiver, and they allow many people with extensive disabilities to avoid the prospect of institutional care. They are also a valuable source of additional support for people who depend on their family and friends for primary care.

Community volunteers cook meals, clean houses, and provide transportation to many activities. Organizations that perform these tasks include Meals on Wheels. Individual volunteers may be students from high schools, colleges, or universities who are required to complete the work as part of their degree program. You may even be able to obtain the support of retired nurses, therapists, and physicians. They can provide invaluable expertise.

Local media outlets frequently support local citizens by conducting fund-raising activities, publicizing discrimination and mistreatment, and increasing public awareness of specific conditions. The media also encourage citizens to contribute to blood banks, organ banks, and volunteer drives.

The Government

Many people with special needs are eligible for government support programs. Care can be expensive, and often your disability will cause at least a temporary loss of income. In these cases, some funding may be available to help meet the costs, and the government can be a valuable source of support. However, the reality is that in most instances, government support is not sufficient to meet the costs associated with disability. Government cutbacks have had a disproportionate impact on people with disabilities and their families, and in the last decade the level of available support has diminished.

Contact a local social worker or doctor to find out what support is available. To access specific programs such as Workers' Compensation, you may require legal advice. Although you should investigate all of these options, remember that thousands of individuals spend hours in fruitless attempts to have all of their needs met by the government. If you can get government support, that is great, but a good personal protection plan will mean you are not at the mercy of government eligibility requirements.

HOW DO I ESTABLISH A SUPPORT NETWORK?

This is a step-by-step guide to building your support network, a process you should start as soon as your disability is diagnosed. If you lack confidence in your ability to build a support network because of your physical condition or your lack of expertise, it may be a good idea to retain the services of an advocate.

1. **Contact the nearest disability-specific support organization.** Many of the support group members will have already established their own support network, and they will be able to give you names, phone numbers, Web sites, and recommendations of personnel. They will also alert you to any pitfalls. They will be able to provide you with a framework modelled on their own experience, which you can either follow or modify to your own experience. This will help you along the way.

2. **Assess available resources.** Once your support group has informed you of the resources that are available in your

community, you will be able to assess how relevant or well-matched each service is to your needs. Once you have assessed these services, you will be able to select the ones that are most appropriate for your needs.

3. **Determine your needs.** Before you approach any organizations with specific requests for help, you should have a clear idea of the areas in which you would most benefit from added support. You should make a list of your financial, medical, physical, and personal needs, and then assess where your care program is most deficient. At that point, you can approach the relevant organizations to see if they can meet your needs. Their experience may lead them to suggest additional areas of concern that you may not have thought of on your own.

4. **Contact relevant parties.** This can be a time-consuming activity, as you may have to write or phone many different organizations and groups in order to build an effective support network. When you call, you should clearly explain who you are, what your condition is, and what type of support you, or your loved one, require. Follow-up letters from physicians, therapists, or other caregivers will provide greater detail and legitimate your needs.

5. **Consult with relevant parties.** Once a group has agreed to work with you, you should invite them to your hospital, rehabilitation facility, or home for an initial assessment. At this assessment, you should go into precise detail about your requirements and schedule so that they can serve you effectively. This exchange provides an opportunity for you to explain your personal preferences and develop a relationship with the volunteers. Once you have sorted out the details, the organizations or individuals can begin to provide you with support.

6. **Develop back-up measures.** Even if you have commitments from caregivers, they may not always come through. Back-up arrangements must always be built in to home care, therapy, transportation, and other services. It is essential that you develop a list of people who are available twenty-four hours a day, seven days a week to meet crisis situations. Often, these people will be your closest friends and family members. In larger communities, professional personnel are available to handle emergencies, but their services may be expensive.

7. **Maintain the network.** Many people over- or underestimate the support they will need. Those who experience degenerative conditions may find that the level of care they need will increase. Therefore, it is important to constantly re-evaluate your needs and make alterations to your support networks on a regular basis.

Edith

Edith was a thirty-eight-year-old, single photographer who became a quadriplegic after a car accident. She spent four months in hospital and six weeks in a rehabilitation centre before she was able to go home. The rehabilitation centre sent a social worker to evaluate Edith's needs and to arrange for a group of caregivers that included physio, occupational, and speech therapists; part-time nursing staff; a Meals on Wheels service; and volunteer students who performed light housekeeping tasks and shopping, and kept Edith company. The centre also arranged for a bus service, which provided transportation to doctors' offices, the local swimming pool, and a twice-weekly social group for individuals with similar conditions. Edith's social worker also contacted the local spinal injuries association, which participated in the provision of these services.

Edith found a great deal of comfort in her social group; she felt at ease with people who had similar medical problems and could empathize with her everyday struggles. She became friends with a number of people in this group, and most of the members motivated each other to become as independent as possible. The spinal injuries association also had an organization for the families of patients, which met on a monthly basis. Members of this group discussed effective caregiving strategies and shared their own stories. They would also debate a case each week to determine how best to provide care. These meetings showed family members a wide range of strategies they could use, and helped them to develop a social network with the other families in the group.

One of the major problems all of these families encountered was that they needed time for rest and relaxation. Some of the families contacted and used professional respite caregivers, and they then referred these supplementary caregivers to the other people in the group who needed their services. They also kept on file the names of three individuals who could come in emergencies or on very short notice to provide supplementary care.

To maintain the support network, Edith and her family continued to attend meetings regularly. At these meetings, they often viewed instructional films or listened to professionals who were brought in to give lectures on relevant topics. Six months after Edith entered the support network, her fellow members were able to arrange a telephone communications hook-up specially adapted for those with spinal injuries and easy for most of the members to access. This allowed members to increase their network of contacts, and quickly make specific requests whenever they were in need.

In this case, a professional social worker was available to lay the groundwork for the support network. People who do not have as much experience in this field may find it difficult to set up a similar system, but they can achieve equally effective results. Even if a professional social worker cannot establish the entire support network, she can provide valuable advice and contact names to point you in the right direction and save you a lot of time. When setting up a support network, make sure that you contact local phone companies and computer specialists to request information on the latest technology, and to push them to provide services that will strengthen your network.

Morry

Morry was a businessman who lived in Atlanta. At the age of thirty-nine, he was diagnosed with multiple sclerosis (MS), a motor neurone disorder that severely hampered his motor skills. Morry spoke to his physician about his condition and went on the Internet to learn more. He was initially overwhelmed by the requirements of his condition, and by the maze of personnel and facilities he needed. But he called his local MS support group within days of being diagnosed, and staff provided him with a set of contact numbers for professionals, caregivers, programs, and equipment in his area. They also gave him the addresses of the best Internet sites on his condition so he could access the most relevant information from across the continent. He read all of the books and Internet material available, and spoke to many of those involved in the assessment and care of people with MS. Having familiarized himself with all of his options, he selected the personnel and support measures that he felt were most appropriate for him, and developed his own network over the course of several months. After he completed this process, he recorded everything he had done in a manual for other people with MS. His guide was transcribed, photocopied, and distributed to other members of his support group.

Once he had successfully established his own support network, he recognized that there was a need in the community for a central organization that could direct people with special needs to the appropriate resources. A year and a half after he was first diagnosed with MS, he created a central clearinghouse to help all people with disabilities create personal support networks. While developing a support network can be a daunting task, anyone with sufficient effort and allies can become an expert!

CUSTOM-DESIGNED PROGRAMS

In many cases, the existing support services will be sufficient to meet your needs, but occasionally you will be required to work with service providers to modify a program to suit your circumstances, or even to design an entirely new program.

How to Design a New Program

Below is a step-by-step process to design a new program, followed by examples for each step:

1. **Determine your needs.** A sixty-two-year-old woman had a stroke and became partially paralysed. She lived in a small community fifteen miles outside of Chicago. Although her neighbours were very supportive, there was no one in the village who had the skills to provide the proper care. Her husband met with a social worker from the city, and they drew up a list of his wife's needs and the requirements of her care. The list included a physiotherapist, nursing care, and a group of volunteers who could stay with the woman while her husband was at work during the week.

2. **Locate suitable personnel.** The husband, in conjunction with the social worker, located people who could provide the necessary care. They found a physiotherapist and nurse who were willing to travel to the village to train the

volunteer caregivers to take care of the woman properly. The husband and the social worker also actively canvassed the village to locate a committed group of approximately twenty-five volunteers who were willing to provide long-term care.

3. **Provide necessary training.** The nurse came in once a week to teach the volunteers how to properly bathe, feed, and medicate their client. She also taught them the danger signs that would indicate the re-occurrence of a stroke or possible cardiac problems, and how to guard against or treat bed sores, which were a recurring problem.

The physiotherapist provided eight of the volunteers with instruction in the exercise program needed to strengthen the patient's right side, which had been severely damaged by the stroke. After three three-hour training sessions, the volunteers were able to provide the therapy that the patient required. These eight volunteers were also able to train the others in their group, so all twenty-five were eventually able to provide adequate physiotherapy. The physiotherapist returned every two weeks to assess the progress of the patient.

4. **Schedule and maintain programming and care.** The social worker, in conjunction with the nurse, the physiotherapist, and the husband, designed a schedule with back-up personnel so the patient's needs would always be met, even when her husband was at work. Because of the generosity of the volunteers in the village, this schedule was easy to establish and maintain. The nurse and physiotherapist continued to visit on a weekly basis for the next sixteen months to ensure the continuity of care. After sixteen months, the woman was rehabilitated to the point where she was able to live without outside assistance.

Living in a Small Community

If you live in a small community, the resources you need may not be available. As a result, you will have to be creative. This may in fact be easier in a small community, where personal relationships are often closer and rates of volunteerism are almost always higher than in big cities. If everybody knows everybody else, people are more comfortable asking for and offering help. In addition, the Internet has lessened the isolation of people living in small communities, and has provided greater access to information and support. In some instances, however, such as when specialized medical treatment or therapy is required, it may be necessary to move to a larger community on a temporary, and sometimes permanent, basis.

Orrin

Orrin was a dairy farmer in Pennsylvania. He was severely injured when his tractor rolled over as he was attempting to plough a section of land with a steep grade. He had a broken leg, and sustained injuries to his neck, back, and shoulders. As a result of his injuries, Orrin was unable to work for a year and a half, and he faced the loss of his property. His wife was taking care of their two young children and could not take over the operation of the farm. Happily, Orrin's friends and neighbours took over the entire operation of his farm during his recuperation, and they were able to avert a potentially tragic situation. Orrin was overwhelmed by this generous show of support. He was fortunate to have such caring and dedicated neighbours.

CONCLUSION

Much like the individual who has the disability, caregivers have to go through an adjustment process. You must accept that life has changed and that you will have to make some new arrangements.

A positive attitude is just as important for caregivers as it is for people living with disabilities. Caregivers have the power to control and shape the changes that disability brings — they can emphasize the positives in any situation. With the proper support, caregivers can help anyone triumph over disability.

8

Maximizing
Medical Care

INTRODUCTION

The people you choose to help you overcome your disability will have a tremendous impact on your physical and mental well-being. The right caregivers can motivate you, help build and maintain your self-esteem, and aid in your adjustment and integration.

Don't allow yourself to be cared for by unqualified or inferior personnel. Care given by people who are not adequately trained can slow your progress, and may even have a negative effect. You have the right to the best care available, and if you are diligent, you should never have to settle for second best. If you make a concerted effort to learn about your condition and the range of treatment options available, you will be able to take control and make the decisions that will ensure that you receive the best possible care.

Sometimes patients have to choose between three or four caregivers or methods of treatment. When there are a number of reasonable options, it can be difficult to make a decision. Educating yourself, consulting with experts, and keeping an open mind will help you to make an appropriate choice. This chapter will guide you through the process of making decisions about medical care: what you should look for, where to look for it, who to go to for help, and how to ensure that you are treated properly. It will explain the skills and qualities you should seek in your caregivers, and the steps you can follow to ensure that you get the most out of your care.

YOUR RELATIONSHIP WITH YOUR CAREGIVERS

Health-care professionals should be allies, not adversaries. The healing process cannot occur in isolation. In order to reach your maximum rehabilitative potential, you must be a fully informed participant in any treatment program. You, the patient, have the only true key to your recovery: motivation. Patient motivation can be encouraged by promoting an egalitarian approach to care, a sort of "team healing" effort. The natural resources of the body can, and indeed must, be mobilized to cope effectively with illness. This requires you to trust your own judgement, and to work co-operatively with medical professionals. You should be seen as the main actor in your own treatment, and the caregiver as your assistants.

Health-care professionals can forget that patients are whole people who think and feel, who possess knowledge, experience, and opinions. Because doctors are essential to care, they sometimes have a tendency to treat their patients as helpless babies who need to be taken care of. The doctors who thrive in this authoritarian role — those who make decisions without consulting their patients, who withhold information, and who ignore patients' wishes — incapacitate their patients. Doctors deserve respect, but they are not deserving of idolatry. Work with medical professionals to amplify your natural self-healing capacities.

MAKING GOOD DECISIONS ABOUT YOUR CARE

To be an effective judge of your therapy programs, you must read extensively and consult physicians, your support group, and other experts. There are several steps you can follow to become an informed and competent consumer of services.

Speak to Your Personal Physician or Specialist

Once you have been diagnosed, your family physician or specialist will help you set the foundation for your care plan and caregiving team. They will be able to suggest the patterns of treatment and the personnel you require. The physician will usually set out a range of options covering areas as diverse as physiotherapy, drug treatment, diet, and others. Don't be overwhelmed, even if you are unfamiliar with the consequences of the choices you have to make. At this point, education is essential.

Educate Yourself About Your Choices

Read as much as you can. Books on your condition, medical journals, and the Internet can all be valuable sources of information. If you are unable to locate what you are looking for, or if you do not have access to some of these resources, ask a local librarian for help. She will provide expert advice that will narrow your search and make it easier to find the information you need. Other people who have made similar choices can also help you to understand the implications of your choices. Talking to someone who has undergone the same surgery or treatments you are considering will provide a perspective that you can't always find in a book. Support groups will be able to give you these contacts.

If your disability has been sudden and you don't have the time or the energy to do the research, a family member or an advocate can do it for you, and can help clarify your options. If you require immediate treatment, you may have no time to investigate your options and will have to rely solely on your physician's advice. You can follow a rational, deliberate, decision-making process after your condition has stabilized. For example, when I had my first heart attack, the attending physician told me, "You are having a heart attack, and you have to take this drug immediately to stop muscle damage. Sign here." I knew nothing about the relative merits or dangers of the drug, but at that time I was scared for my life. I had no choice but to trust the doctor. The drug worked, minimizing the damage to my heart.

Don't Be Afraid to Ask for a Second Opinion

If you are uncomfortable with your diagnosis, or with the treatment options your doctor has provided, don't be afraid to ask for a second opinion. Some doctors may be upset if you challenge their judgement, but your satisfaction and confidence in your care program are most important. Another doctor may be able to provide new insights or a more innovative treatment.

Sometimes doctors have to tell you bad news, and it is a natural inclination to ask for a second opinion. If a second doctor confirms your diagnosis, it is worthwhile to focus on maximizing your care program. Doing something to overcome the bad news is often a better policy than trying to find a doctor who will tell you what you want to hear.

It can also be a good idea to avoid taking good news at face value. When I had my first heart attack, the doctors in emergency took great care of me and helped save my life. Afterwards, when I was recovering in the hospital, they told me how fortunate I was that there was only limited damage to my heart. After a couple of weeks, they sent me home with a restricted diet, a personalized exercise program, and five different medications. I felt a great sense of relief. I believed that my heart was in good shape, and that I was going to be okay.

Two weeks later, I felt very ill and experienced angina, the chest pain that often follows a heart attack. I was re-admitted to the hospital, and blood tests revealed that I had just had a second heart attack. I remained in the hospital for a couple of weeks until I finally had an angiogram (a test to reveal blockages in the heart's arteries). The tests indicated that two of my arteries were completely blocked. These blockages did not occur between my first and second heart attacks. When I was sent home after my first heart attack, I was literally a walking time bomb.

I should have been fully tested after my first heart attack, but I was so happy when the doctors told me my heart was okay that I did not think to ask for an angiogram to reveal if my arteries were blocked. I accepted the doctors' directives because I was hoping for the best, and the physicians released me because they thought that I had only minor, temporary damage. It is the patient's responsibility to confirm a diagnosis. If you or your guardians fail to ask the right questions, you may be at greater risk for inappropriate treatment.

It was only later on in my recovery that I was able to learn more about heart disease and begin taking an active role in decisions about my care. Sometimes the information you learn can be intimidating ("You mean you're really going to stop my heart for half an hour?"), but staying focused on your goals can help you overcome any squeamishness. Once you are aware of your options, trust yourself to make an informed decision.

Evaluate Caregivers

Always evaluate the qualifications and reputations of the personnel who treat you. This means confirming your physician's area or areas of expertise, her training, her membership in professional organizations, and her position in a clinic or other treatment centre. Support groups and other patients may provide help in developing an assessment.

Evaluate Treatments

There are a number of important questions you can ask your physician, other medical specialists, or other people who have had your condition that can help you to evaluate your treatment options.

- Are there side effects? If so, what are they?
- How painful is the therapy?
- What will this treatment cost me?
- What is my full range of options?
- Are you aware of any viable experimental treatments?
- How often have you done this procedure?
- What decisions have other patients with my condition made?
- What outcomes did they experience?
- How does my age affect the prognosis?
- Will this treatment affect my existing medical conditions?
- What is the best that I can hope for?
- How much time will the procedure take?
- What can I do to make the treatment most effective?

Going through this list of questions, plus any others you think of before you initiate surgery or treatment, will enhance your understanding of what you will go through and help focus your decision-making.

Check the Caregiver's Reputation

If you require specialized treatment, a doctor will often give you a list of several practitioners, along with her recommendation. While your doctor will usually provide you with good advice, the best way to supplement her advice is by interviewing the candidates and some patients who have undergone similar treatment. Many medical specialists have tight schedules, so you may have to rely on their reputations and your discussions with other patients. Some hospitals also publish the number of surgeries and success rates of various surgeons, which can be a helpful guide.

Organize Your Thoughts

Making a chart rating the caregivers will help you organize your thoughts and will allow you to compare caregivers more easily. Over time, your needs or your assessment of the caregivers may change, so it is important to evaluate your personnel continually and to make sure that you are getting the best possible care.

CRITERIA FOR SELECTING THE APPROPRIATE PERSONNEL

Although caregivers perform many different functions, there are some characteristics all of them should possess. These criteria can serve as a guide for your evaluation.

Ethical Standards

All caregivers are expected to follow professional standards of conduct, as set out by their professional regulatory body. They should also acknowledge your freedom of choice in the selection of medical or rehabilitative programs, and commit to providing you with appropriate and compassionate care.

Respect

Caregivers should always respect and appreciate your values and opinions. If you are treated with respect, you will feel more secure and confident in your caregiver. If your caregiver treats you as a partner *with* whom they work, rather than a case *on* which they work, you will be motivated to play a greater role in your own rehabilitation.

Flexibility

A physician or caregiver should always be willing to examine new or unique programs of treatment. The early adoption of a therapy on the cutting edge can make a significant difference in your well-being. There is also the possibility, however, that an experimental treatment may be harmful to your health. Another drawback is that some medical plans do not cover experimental treatments. Whenever possible, try to strike a balance between traditional and innovative therapies.

Physicians who recommend innovative treatments are usually well informed about your disease or disability and the risks associated with your pattern of care. If your specialist does not want to proceed with experimental therapy, it is important that at the very least she be made aware of its existence. Alert your doctors if you hear of any new procedures that may prove beneficial. Almost all specialists look after a large number of patients with a range of different conditions, and they may not have the time to keep up to date on the latest innovations for every condition that they treat. For example, if you have an uncommon form of cancer and are constantly on the lookout for information on new treatments, you may read or hear about a procedure before your specialist. A qualified professional will appreciate the information, and should at the very least take the time to evaluate the treatment.

Honesty and Openness About Treatment

Your caregivers, particularly your physicians, should always provide you with detailed information about the care they will provide, as well as an estimate of the cost of the options they recommend. Professionals should be honest about the merits and shortcomings (including side-effects) of any suggested therapies or prescriptions, and, when appropriate, they should inform you of the available alternatives.

Sometimes professionals may inject their biases into their recommendations for treatment. For example, female cancer specialists and surgeons have often been reluctant to recommend complete breast removal for clients who have breast cancer, preferring instead to recommend chemotherapy, radiation therapy, lumpectomies, or partial mastectomies. Male surgeons have been more inclined to recommend full mastectomies. Both strategies can be effective, but you should remember that physicians' opinions are not always objective truths; they are a combination of their education, training, and personal biases. You must sort out the details for yourself, and ensure that the final decision on your care is one with which you are comfortable.

Some professionals believe that they can automatically assume decision-making power over you and prescribe all of the directives you must follow. Adults with disabilities are often treated as objects or cases, rather than as human beings who are rational, intelligent, and have minds of their own. Professionals have skills and powers that you do not possess, but that does not mean you should be excluded from the decision-making process.

Time Management

Scheduling and time management are important considerations when dealing with professionals. They sometimes overbook appointments, or are called on to respond to emergencies, delaying your appointment. To avoid these problems, book well in advance. Whenever possible, call ahead on the day of the appointment to see if there will be any delays. You can adjust your schedule accordingly. Another strategy is to book the first appointment of the day. That way, no one can keep you waiting.

Make sure that the expert you choose will be able to give you the time and commitment you deserve. Some specialists may be too involved with other considerations to provide you with an appropriate level of care. For example, a specialist may have an extraordinary patient load that prevents her from committing the time necessary to provide the proper care. In such a case, you may be well advised to seek out other personnel.

Expertise

All medical specialists will be qualified in their chosen field, but some individuals truly provide leading-edge treatment. A doctor who is a leader in her field may be able to make a difference in your treatment by constantly providing the most advanced care. A doctor's reputation is often a very good guide to the quality of care they will provide.

When I was eighteen years old, a good friend of mine was diagnosed with leukemia. In 1957 a diagnosis like that was almost always fatal. But Frank's physician, a recent graduate from Yale medical school, had spent the past two summers working with his professor on the latest treatments. He used methods that no other doctor in Calgary had yet learned. With the benefit of his doctor's training and experience, Frank was able to beat the leukemia. He is now the proud father of four children, and he claims he is quite certain that he will die of something else. Physicians who are experts in their field can often achieve miraculous results.

Placing Your Interests First

Doctors and other caregivers should always focus on your well-being, rather than on finding a pattern of treatment that is most cost-effective. This problem is most apparent in Health Maintenance Organizations (HMOs), where the profit motive of the organization can discourage doctors from providing you with the best treatment that is available. Most physicians will make decisions with your best interests in mind, but some care-givers are influenced by financial concerns and other factors, which can lead them to select a pattern of treatment that may not be optimal. Knowledge about your condition can prevent your interests from being compromised. If you are unaware of your options, however, you will be hard-pressed to differentiate between levels of care.

When he could no longer use crutches to move around because of extreme pain in his knee, a seventy-two-year-old man was directed to use a wheelchair by his HMO physician. The doctor gave his patient some painkillers, but advised him that knee-replacement surgery would be inadvisable because he had had a heart attack and single-bypass surgery. The pain in his knee became so extreme that while visiting another city, the man saw his brother's physician for a second opinion. The second doctor informed him that there was no medical reason why he should not have knee-replacement surgery, which would make a big difference in his quality of life.

The man went back to his HMO physician, who was adamant in his refusal to provide the surgery. He was forced to visit a specialist in a clinic not covered by his HMO, where surgery and rehabilitation were provided. The knee replacement was entirely successful and the man was subsequently able to walk with an agility that he had not had in years. He is currently suing his HMO for failing to provide the surgery, and for forcing him to endure a long period of immobility as a result of a diagnosis that could have been motivated by cost-cutting strategies at the HMO.

Participation in Research Projects

It may be worthwhile to consider participating in a research project in order to try experimental therapies that would not otherwise be available. Being part of a research project may help you avoid some of the costs associated with treatment, and you may also benefit from closer medical scrutiny. On the other hand, some medical practitioners may consider you to be little more than a guinea pig. In such a situation, you would be well advised to seek out other personnel.

Compatibility

Some professionals are dictatorial, abrupt, or even rude, and many work under heavy pressure and tight schedules. You have the right to be treated in a fair and courteous manner. If you are not treated appropriately, express your dissatisfaction in a polite yet firm manner to the offending individual. Some professionals are not even aware that their actions are causing you stress, and they will often make an effort to address your concerns after they have been made aware. If you are uncomfortable with confronting them directly, it may be helpful to have a friend, relative, or other caregiver intervene on your behalf. If these interventions do not produce a satisfactory response, consider approaching your caregiver's supervisor with your concerns, or look into switching caregivers. If you do not take any steps to address a personality conflict, it can escalate.

You may have to tolerate an impersonal or rude professional to benefit from her expertise. If this is your only option, try to focus on the benefits you will receive from her experience, rather than on the unpleasant personal side of your relationship. Some professionals place heavy demands on their patients, which can lead to resentment. For example, many rehabilitation therapists push their clients to tremendous levels of pain in order to achieve effective results. Do not confuse a demanding caregiver with a rude or abusive one. Some patients come to resent their therapists, and in extreme cases develop an intense personal dislike for the person who is making them work so hard. In the long run, however, most patients, after seeing the progress they have made, come to realize the contribution of the intense and demanding counsellor to their well-being.

If you believe you would be better off working with different personnel, consult other patients and advocates, who can suggest more personable caregivers. Changing doctors, however, is not a decision to be taken lightly. If at all possible, try to work out your differences with your original physician. Making a change because of incompetence should be done immediately. Making a change because of a personality conflict should be done only as a last resort.

HOW TO GET THE MOST OUT OF YOUR CARE
Once you have decided on the course of action you want to pursue, you can use a number of techniques to safeguard the quality of your care.

Speak Out
Sometimes, people with disabilities have to force doctors, therapists, and even family members to listen to them. Often, caregivers will treat you as a passive participant and categorize

you according to your condition. They may not make a serious effort to respond to your concerns.

You can overcome this problem by establishing your credibility and your right to make important decisions about your care. This can be done by showing that you are knowledgeable about your condition. As an adult, you have the right to control most aspects of your care as long as you are mentally competent. It is a matter of making your voice heard.

Gaining respect from your caregivers is not accomplished by shouting or insisting that you are right all the time. Develop a relationship based on mutual respect. By identifying and expressing any difficulties or reactions you have to drugs or therapies, and by asking pertinent questions, you can convince caregivers that you are interested and involved in your care.

For example, some prescriptions have a positive effect over the short run, but lose their effectiveness with extended exposure. In the wrong combinations, some drugs may even become toxic. By paying close attention to your reactions, you can help your physician find the right pharmaceutical combination. He will appreciate the active role you have taken and become more receptive to your future input.

Ian worked as a retail manager for a chain clothing store in New York. Clinical depression ran in his family, and he was aware of the warning signs. In his mid-twenties, he started experiencing extreme fatigue, he lost his temper easily, he felt nauseated, and he was deeply depressed. He went to a psychiatrist, who prescribed Zoloft, a drug that is commonly used to treat depression. For the first sixth months, the Zoloft was very effective and it eliminated the symptoms of his depression. He did suffer one major side-effect, however: he experienced inorgasmia, a significant problem for a young, single man. But he was willing to tolerate the side-effect in exchange for the drug's benefits. After six months, he began to feel depressed again and discussed these feelings with his psychiatrist, who recommended an increase in dosage. Initially, the increased dosage was effective, but every six months the effects of the Zoloft would wear off. After two years, he was taking four times the original dosage, and he was frustrated with its side-effects. After consulting with his psychiatrist, he decided to switch to Prozac, another antidepressant, which is working effectively and has not caused any major side-effects.

Your wishes will usually be honoured, but some people may have to be forced to listen to you. The best way to ensure that your requests are respected is to legally state them in a power of attorney. For example, an elderly woman with significant financial means wanted to live in her own apartment supported by caregivers twenty-four hours a day. Her family had reservations because this form of care would diminish their inheritance. To protect their inheritance, her children tried to have their ninety-two-year-old mother institutionalized, which would have cost much less. This woman's power of attorney stated that she was to remain independent — she was not to be institutionalized under any circumstances. Her lawyer intervened on her behalf to ensure that her wishes were respected. He explained to the family that he had the ultimate responsibility to carry out his client's wishes, and that her money was designated to provide for her independent care, not to add to their inheritance. As a result, they ceased their legal action.

Explore a Wide Range of Medical Options

Homeopathy, naturopathy, chiropractics, acupuncture, Eastern medicine, and herbal remedies may all be appropriate treatments for your condition. They can help to alleviate pain, enhance rehabilitation, and sometimes even cure you completely. Bonnie

Sherr Klein, a noted author, filmmaker, and activist, has used a wide variety of these therapies to help her overcome two strokes. Once, a doctor asked her, "If you are using all of these techniques, how will you know which one worked?" Klein replied, "Who cares?" You should focus on what makes you feel better, even if you can't identify the specific impact of each element of your care.

While alternative medicines can be very effective, you should always be wary of "snake oil salesmen." Although most practitioners of alternative medicine are legitimate, there are still a large number of con artists who take advantage of people who are concerned about their health. Health fraud is a billion-dollar industry. In the southern United States, for example, many cancer patients went to a private clinic that charged thousands of dollars for a "miracle cure" involving a chemical derived from human urine. The clinic was shut down when health authorities determined that the treatment had no medical value, but not before millions of dollars had been thrown away.

When people fear for their health or their lives, they are at their most vulnerable. Individuals facing death or disability must be wary of falling prey to the false hope offered by cynical profiteers.

Involve Your Family and Closest Friends
In the chapters on caregiving and coping in the family, we discussed the importance of your family and friends. They also have a role to play in ensuring the effectiveness of your medical treatment. Their vigilance can enhance any level of professional care.

Show Appreciation
If you have worked with a caregiver for a long time and appreciate her efforts, let her know how you feel. Thank-you notes, birthday presents, and Christmas gifts tell caregivers that their

efforts are making a difference. If you build a genuine personal relationship with your caregiver, she will often be willing to go that extra mile to help you out.

Keep Accurate Records

During each appointment, take notes that will help you maintain a regular diary of the care you receive. Note your short- and long-term reactions to medical treatments, therapy, drugs, and other interventions. Also, maintain a list of all the treatments you have undergone, so you can evaluate the success of each one. Having an up-to-date list of all your medications is very important, as some drugs react negatively when used in combination with others. This information should be charted in an organized manner so you and your caregivers will be able to evaluate your medical care on an ongoing basis. This is particularly important if you change therapists.

If you always use the same pharmacist, it will be easier for her to keep track of all prescribed medications. If you are seeing several specialists, however, or if you change pharmacists, you must maintain a chart of your own drugs and diet so your medical caregivers do not accidentally prescribe a combination of drugs that may be harmful to you. Doctors will be more receptive to a request to change medication if you give them a detailed list of your drugs and reactions, rather than vague assertions that "the current treatment is making me ill."

Take Appropriate Precautions

If you have allergies, it may be appropriate to wear a Medic Alert bracelet. This piece of jewellery identifies your condition, and shows what triggers the allergies. Medic Alert bracelets can be helpful in emergencies, when you may not be available to provide this information. If you experience noticeable reactions after eating specific foods or ingesting certain drugs, it is imperative that you seek medical attention. Reactions that seem minor today may subsequently become more severe. Traces of seafood in a sauce or peanut oil on a potato chip can cause a severe reaction or even death. If your family has a history of allergies, you should be able to find out if you are at risk. If you or a relative has experienced negative reactions from drugs, medications, or anesthetics, it may indicate the presence of a potentially dangerous condition. This can be confirmed by a doctor.

My neighbour Judith wears a Medic Alert bracelet which indicates that she is allergic to penicillin. If she ever suffers an infection or cut and is unconscious, medical personnel will know not to give her penicillin, which could be fatal. My wife and sons wear Medic Alert bracelets to alert doctors to the possibility that they may have malignant hyperthermia, an allergic reaction to certain anesthetics. These simple precautions save lives.

Maintain Access to Information

Sometimes doctors feel it is appropriate to withhold negative diagnoses. If you want to be fully informed about your condition, regardless of the prognosis, tell your doctor explicitly and incorporate this directive into a living will and power of attorney. These documents will ensure that you are party to all information. Some people, on the other hand, trust their physicians to convey only appropriate information.

A physician will usually withhold information when she feels that the shock of the diagnosis would have a negative effect far outweighing the benefit of complete knowledge. In these instances, doctors usually tell other family members without telling the patient. For example, a physician may not tell an eighty-nine-year-old woman with a heart condition that she has incurable cancer, for fear of inducing a heart attack. Too much knowledge can also sometimes be intimidating. Before my heart surgery, I read a number of articles and books that described the exact procedure of double-bypass surgery. In retrospect, I wish I had not done so, because it served only to increase my anxiety. It was important to be informed about the general details of my upcoming surgery, but the "gory" physical details were intimidating. The amount of information to be shared is a matter of personal choice.

MAKING DIFFICULT DECISIONS

You will not always have weeks or months in which to make a decision. Sometimes your course of care must be decided within hours, if not minutes. If you are seriously injured and require life-saving surgery that may result in incapacitation, you must make a life-altering decision within minutes. Sometimes you may not be capable of making a decision at all. The best way to ensure that your desires are followed is to have a living will and a power of attorney. These documents can provide your answers to a number of difficult questions:

- Do I want to be kept on a respirator?
- Am I willing to lose a limb?
- Would I consider a transplant?
- How long should I be kept on life support?
- Should I donate my organs?
- Will I accept experimental treatment?
- What price am I willing to pay for my life?

It is not always easy to make decisions about your life and health in a period of crisis. Considering the key issues beforehand can assure you that you have made the correct decision.

You also have the right to refuse treatment. Not all people want to extend their lives for as long as possible; some are primarily concerned with quality-of-life issues. What constitutes quality of life will vary from person to person. If you believe you know what your decision would be if you were faced with intubation or severe pain, then a power of attorney or a living will can ensure that there is no confusion. Review these documents on a regular basis to ensure that you still agree with your stated decisions.

YOUR RESPONSIBILITIES TO YOUR CAREGIVERS

Although your caregiver is there to work for you, it is not a one-way street. If you acknowledge and fulfil your responsibilities to your caregiver, your level of care will be improved.

Take Responsibility

Caregivers sometimes encounter patients who are uninformed or unwilling to make difficult decisions. This places an added responsibility on the caregiver, who in most cases should only recommend courses of action, not choose them. This scenario is common in seniors' residences. Some patients are unwilling to enter a nursing home or hire the necessary support staff, even though they are unable to take care of themselves. In this situation, an attendant is required to provide a level of care that is beyond her capacity to deliver. The caregiver will be forced to inform her supervisors that she can no longer provide care, which can create significant tensions between the patient, her family, the caregivers, and the institution. Sometimes the intervention of social services is required to resolve these difficulties. To avoid similar problems, you should be prepared to make difficult decisions. Be realistic in appraising your needs and choices.

Ruth

I worked with Ruth, an eighty-five-year-old widow whose mind was very sharp, but who had a number of physical problems, including arthritis, high blood pressure, and obesity. With the assistance of full-time attendants, she remained in her own home for eight years. Eventually, her caregivers claimed that Ruth was too heavy for them to provide the safe, high-level nursing care that she needed. The caregivers found it very hard to lift Ruth, which created problems with bathing, toileting, and other areas of personal care. Some caregivers sustained back and neck injuries, and one dislocated his shoulder lifting Ruth out of the bathtub.

The caregivers told Ruth and her family that they could not provide competent care on a long-term basis, and that she should enter a hospital or long-term care facility. Ruth was fiercely independent, however, and refused to enter these institutions under any circumstances. Nine different caregivers worked with Ruth over a two-month period, and each one worked for an average of just three weeks before leaving. The caregivers would call Ruth's family and say that they were not coming in to work because it was an impossible situation. Her family members would then have to come in and provide care, disrupting their day-to-day responsibilities. Ruth's sense of independence was admirable, but her unwillingness to recognize that she was not safe at home created havoc for everyone.

Do Your Share

It is a physician's responsibility to treat you with consideration and compassion, but you must also accept responsibility for your care. Once you have established a pattern of care, it is in your interests to follow the program closely. Make every effort to take your medication as prescribed and follow your rehabilitation schedule and diet plan. If you do not uphold your end of the bargain, your care will suffer. Recognize that you are not your doctor's only patient, and understand that he also has demands placed on his time. Make the effort to be on time for your appointments and to be prepared when you meet.

Keep Your Cool

Patients occasionally take out their frustrations on their caregivers. Although this is inappropriate, it occurs on a regular basis. Try to discuss your frustrations with counsellors instead of lashing out at them. If you do get angry and shout at a caregiver, it is not the end of the world. Nurses, doctors, and therapists are all trained professionals who realize that their patients are under stress. If you are willing to apologize for losing your cool, and you make an effort to treat the caregiver with respect, you will be able to overcome any temporary conflicts and continue working together.

My father was very angry about losing a leg when he was eighty-one years old. The frustration of relearning how to walk and living with the phantom pain in his amputated leg caused him to lash out at his caregivers. One wonderful friend who took my father on many day trips set him straight after he had yelled at him without good reason. Eric told my dad that he had to grow up, and that if he ever swore in his company again, Eric would never return for another visit. He went on to warn my father to moderate his behaviour or risk losing many of his friends and his caregivers. From then on, my dad was able to manage his temper and treat his caregivers with the respect they deserved.

PERSONNEL CHART

The following chart can help you keep track of some of the personnel you may consult over the course of your care.

Medical and Paramedical Personnel	Address and Contact Number	Comments
Physicians: General Practitioner Specialist Psychiatrist		
Psychologists		
Dentists		
Nurses Nurses' Aides		
Therapists: Physiotherapist Occupational Therapist Speech Therapist Rehabilitation Therapist		
Counsellors		
Audiologists		
Personal Attendants		
Public Support Personnel	**Address and Contact Number**	**Comments**
Social Workers		
Intervenors		
Government Employees: Local, State or Provincial Federal		
Appeal Boards		
Other Resources	**Address and Contact Number**	**Comments**
Service Clubs		
Community Groups		
Charities and Foundations		
Advocacy Groups		
Support Groups		
Disability Groups		

CONCLUSION

Organizing and evaluating your care is an essential ingredient in developing an effective plan. You are the one who should have ultimate control over your care, but you will need the expertise of medical and paramedical personnel to rehabilitate to your maximum potential. If you are aware of the positive qualities to look for in a caregiver, and are able to marshall your resources, you will be able to get the most out of your medical care.

Chapter

9

Avoiding Stress
and Burnout

INTRODUCTION

Stress results from the pressures you can encounter at work, in
your social life, from a disability, or from any other issue. Stress
can have positive or negative consequences, depending on how
you respond to it. You can react to a stressful situation by working
harder to overcome the source of stress, or you can let it get you
down. Throughout this book, we have emphasized the importance of having a positive attitude, planning in advance, and
taking control of your situation. These strategies will help you
use stress to your advantage.

Allowing stress to build up can place you at risk of burnout.
Burnout occurs when you simply can't take it any more — when
the strain of caregiving and of all the other pressures in your life
combine to make it seem like you can't go on. People who suffer
from burnout are at a greater risk of alcoholism, depression, and
family breakdown, and they may abuse the people in their care.

The people most at risk from burnout are the ones who try to do everything on their own. Without support from family, friends, or support groups, they have no one to relieve them when times get tough. If you approach the stresses of caregiving within a framework of support, you can manage the consequences of stress and avoid burnout.

The first step towards building this framework is to recognize that you can't do everything on your own. Be ready to bring in outside resources to help you cope. The second step is to identify possible sources of stress, and be ready for them. After your stressors have been identified, you can then select the strategies you will use to overcome them.

Jack and Bill

Jack was a forty-five-year-old mechanic with a wife, Helen, and three children. His brother Bill, who worked as a stockbroker, went through a messy divorce. Bill's wife was awarded their home and custody of their two children. Bill's work began to suffer as a result of his family problems, and he lost his job. Shortly afterwards, Bill had a nervous breakdown. After being treated in the hospital for six weeks, Bill left the institution. Jack offered to take his brother in.

Bill decided to move in with his brother's family. In the first month he was there he made numerous attempts to find a new position in the financial services industry, but he was unsuccessful. Bill's inability to find work made him depressed and angry.

He placed several demands on Jack and his family. He demanded a special diet because he was a vegetarian, and he did not like to be left alone at night, "because he had fears of being attacked by his creditors." Most of the time Bill got along well with the children, but sometimes he would become very upset when they made noise, which he claimed "disturbed his thinking."

Helen defended her children when Bill yelled at them, which made for several ugly confrontations. She grew concerned about the distress he was causing the children. As Bill's inability to find work dragged on, he became more irritable and began to chain smoke. His bursts of anger became more frequent, and Jack noticed that Bill would have difficulty focusing during conversation. Jack and Helen became more reluctant to have people over when Bill was at home.

Arguments within the family became more frequent as Bill's demands and erratic behaviour increased. Helen and Jack began to argue about him. Helen suggested that they may have to ask Bill to leave because of the disruption he was causing. Jack stood up for his brother, who had nowhere else to go, though his own work and health were starting to suffer. Jack and Helen decided that there would have to be changes if Bill was going to continue to live with them.

Jack and Helen visited Bill's psychiatrist to discuss the strategies they could use to make their living arrangements easier. They described the deterioration in Bill's condition, and the problems that they were having. The psychiatrist suggested that Bill's behaviour indicated he was not taking his medication on a regular basis. She recommended that Jack join a support group for families of people with mental illness. She also recommended that they return the next week, with Bill, to establish a "living plan."

The next week, Jack, Helen, and Bill met with the psychiatrist. Jack and Helen told Bill that although they loved him, if he wanted to continue living with their family he would have to take his medication every day and find a job, even if it weren't in his chosen field. Bill would also have to join Jack and Helen in the support group. He would have to assume added responsibilities around the house, and agree not to vent his anger at the children.

Bill accepted these terms, and everyone agreed to start over with a clean slate. He started by quitting smoking and renewing his efforts to find employment. He was successful a few weeks later. He began writing a column on investments for a community paper, and one of his friends found him a part-time job completing tax returns and doing other accounting work for a small firm. He took his medication regularly, even though it would occasionally cause nausea.

Bill began visiting his children again, and re-established relationships with many of the friends he had avoided following his breakdown. He began to pay rent, and he established new friendships with people from work and his support group.

Jack and Helen made an extra effort to resume their former lifestyle. They invited more friends over to their home, and they resumed their habit of jogging together every morning before work. The decision to organize arrangements in the household and set strict criteria that everyone would have to abide by alleviated the major stresses that had developed.

For the next six months, everything went smoothly in the household. Bill was able to save some money, which enabled him to move into an apartment of his own. His family's assistance and intervention were essential in allowing him to start over.

SIGNS OF STRESS

Everyone has bad days. No one can be at their happiest or most optimistic all the time. You are not necessarily facing unmanageable levels of stress every time you have an argument or get upset. Look instead for long-term patterns of behaviour. Persistent feelings of irritation, depression, anxiety, insomnia, and over-aggressiveness, as well as verbal or physical abuse, are signs of mismanaged stress. They should serve as a warning.

SOURCES OF STRESS

We have grouped the most common sources of stress for people with disabilities and their caregivers into three categories: interpersonal stress, medical stress, and other sources of stress. We describe each type, and provide general strategies for beating them.

Interpersonal Stress

These are the stresses that will emerge as a result of your everyday interactions with friends, family, caregivers, or even strangers.

Personal Stress

This stress is caused by the shock of diagnosis and the challenges of living with a disability. Personal stress includes the pressures that you put on yourself. All other forms of stress can be considered components of personal stress.

Stress Within the Family

This is created when anxiety builds up between family members. The pressures of caregiving, changing roles, and new responsibilities can all contribute to family stress.

Stress Between Partners

Any relationship has its ups and downs. This type of stress results from emotional and sexual issues, as well as from the everyday disagreements and pressures that exist in any relationship.

Stress with Caregivers

Spending time with the same person day after day can lead to an accumulation of small grievances that boil over, or larger disagreements about patterns of care.

Stress of Advocacy Roles
When you engage in advocacy, you are often involved in intense personal interactions. Extended attempts to achieve success can be very stressful.

Stress of Social Pressures
The way that friends, family members, and strangers perceive you can change following a disability. Disability can also place constraints on your social life. Adapting to changes in your social situation can cause stress.

Medical Stress
Medical stress is what you experience in relation to your medical care.

Stress of Diagnosis
Some disabilities are difficult to diagnose, and when you finally get the news it can be traumatic, even if you have been expecting negative results. This type of stress results when you are trying to adjust to a diagnosis.

Stress of Pain
Medication cannot always alleviate severe or chronic pain. Living with this pain causes physical and psychological stress.

Stress of Potentially Terminal Condition
A potentially terminal diagnosis can lead to questions about your mortality, and about how your family will cope without you. Facing death is obviously stressful.

Stress of Ongoing Tests and Treatment
Many disabilities require ongoing treatments that can last years and even decades. The constant grind of these therapies can cause stress.

Stress with Medical Personnel
Personality conflicts with medical personnel and other caregivers can detract from the quality of your care and cause stress.

Stress of Unknown Outcomes
The long-term outcome of many diseases and disabilities is unknown. This uncertainty can lead to an increase in personal stress and an accumulation of tension between family members.

Other Sources of Stress
This is a broad, catch-all category.

Stress of Waiting
This is the tension you feel while waiting for doctors, tests, diagnosis, and treatment.

Stress of Disappointment
Not all treatments or therapies are successful. When one of your programs fails, it can be very disappointing and can affect how you approach other issues.

Decision-Making Stress
Individuals often have to make very difficult decisions over the course of their disability. When you have to choose a caregiving strategy that will make a big difference in your life, the pressure of making the right choice can be stressful.

Financial Stress
The costs that can emerge from a disability can put a strain on a family's resources. Constantly worrying about finding the money to pay for treatment and even basic expenses can create stress for everyone involved.

Stress of Relocation
If you need to be close to a specific medical facility or specialist, you may have to move. Relocating away from your friends or family can be stressful.

Stress of Adapting to a Permanent Disability
Adapting to an amputation or other permanent condition often requires a re-evaluation of self-image and goals.

GENERAL STRATEGIES FOR COPING WITH STRESS

There are a number of basic strategies that can help you cope with all forms of stress.

- **Engage in regular physical activity.** Regular physical activities such as walking, swimming, jogging, yoga, t'ai chi, or any of your favourite sports can help to relieve the physical symptoms of stress.
- **Maintain a healthy lifestyle.** It is important to maintain a healthy diet and get the rest, relaxation, and sleep that you require. When you become fatigued and run down, you are more vulnerable to stress.
- **Everything in moderation.** Avoid dependence on drugs, alcohol, and tobacco. They can exacerbate chronic conditions and hinder rehabilitation. Any kind of chemical dependence will decrease the quality of care over the long term.

- **Focus on other interests.** If disability becomes the only concern in your life, it can cause mental fatigue. Try not to think about it twenty-four hours a day. Engage in your favourite leisure activities, go out for a nice dinner, read a book, or go to a concert. Consider taking continuing education courses or developing new hobbies and skills.
- **Maintain your social life.** Set aside time to go out with your friends. Caregiving is a major responsibility, but you won't be effective if you neglect your own need for fun, laughter, and companionship.
- **Take time for yourself every day.** Taking a small time-out every day can make a big difference. It can help you put your challenges in perspective, and allow you to approach them slightly refreshed each day.
- **Assess and adjust.** It is important to evaluate your situation constantly so that you can identify and make changes to your lifestyle or care plan. If your needs change, it can mean that some of your coping strategies won't work any more. However, if you are closely attuned to your care, a simple adjustment will be all that is needed to address many of your problems.
- **Relax!** Caregiving can be a high-stress occupation, but you can't fire on all cylinders all of the time. Sometimes you have to force yourself to relax. Set aside time each day for a nap or for a fifteen- or thirty-minute period in which you will not worry. Meditation is an excellent way to practise relaxation and calm yourself down.
- **Organize care.** Managing your time and organizing your environment is a central part of any overall strategy for dealing with stress. Prioritize your tasks. Emphasize those that are most important, and that require innovation and experimentation, and de-emphasize, delegate, or eliminate

those that are trivial and routine. You must also learn how to say no. Resist needless draws on your time. It is okay to refuse an invitation or a request for something if you need to focus on your own well-being or your caregiving role.

- **Be proactive.** Don't just sit around stewing because a problem exists. Figure out what you can do to change it.

Coping with Interpersonal Stress

It is essential to engage in open and honest communication with your family members and caregivers. These strategies can help you cope with interpersonal stress:

- Have weekly discussions in which everyone can feel free to discuss their concerns in an open, non-judgemental environment.
- Talk about problems as soon as they arise. Small problems can grow into big ones if they are not addressed immediately. Don't allow issues to fester.
- Don't keep your emotions bottled up inside. Share your stress with members of your support group. That's what they are there for.
- Give and demand respect. Respect is a two-way street. You cannot expect people to treat you with respect if you do not extend them the same courtesy.
- Engage in counselling. Some interpersonal problems need a third person to mediate them, or to provide a new perspective. Trained counsellors can help you resolve conflicts that you could not manage on your own.

Coping with Medical Stress

Here is a list of strategies to help you cope with medical stress:

- Build a solid relationship with your caregivers through the strategies described in Chapter 8. Participating in your own care gives you confidence and control over your situation. When you feel in control, stress is minimized.
- Make a list and put each of your stressors into one of two categories: Things I Can Control and Things I Can't Control. Take steps to address everything you can control, and try not to worry too much about the things you can't. If there is something you want to gain control over that is beyond your command right now, discuss the issue with your caregivers or an expert. You may be able to change things from one category to another.
- Define your quality-of-life objectives and adjust your medical plan accordingly. Don't accept a treatment plan that is not in line with your priorities. Medical care is about healing your whole person, not just the part of you that is "sick." Don't accept an unsatisfactory treatment plan.
- Turn uncertainty into a positive. Not knowing how your condition will progress can serve as a motivating factor. Because the outcome is uncertain, you have the opportunity to change it. By channelling your uncertainty into hard work, you can make the stress a positive stress.

Coping with Other Stresses

- **Be prepared to improvise.** Don't adhere to a routine or a treatment just because it is the routine. If something isn't working, don't give up. Consult with your caregivers and try something else.

- **Redefine your goals.** If disability changes your abilities, you can set new goals that take into account what you can do, not what you used to be able to do. Your goals should reflect what you can accomplish, not societal standards of success.
- **Have confidence.** No matter how hard the choices become, be assured that you know yourself best. If you have educated yourself about your condition, be satisfied that you will make the right decision. Don't worry about choices you have made in the past. If you make a mistake, learn from it and move on, don't wallow in regret. If you are uncertain about a particular decision, there are always resources available to guide you through your options.
- **Know your limitations.** Push as hard as you can, but know when to draw the line. If you are constantly exhausted, your health may suffer.
- **Be ready for "old" stresses.** Disability will not bring an end to the stresses you faced in your job, or around politics, the environment, or your favourite baseball team. When these stresses arise, treat them just as you did before — as everyday bumps in a road that you can handle.
- **Prioritize.** People who experience significant disabilities often radically reorganize their priorities. This can be one of the major positives of a disabling experience. Something that was a huge issue before may no longer seem important. Some stresses will cause you problems only if you let them.
- **Emphasize what you have, not what you don't have.** Sometimes you may be faced with very unappealing choices. Being confronted with the possible amputation of your leg is an example of this. In such a situation, focusing on the rehabilitation you will undertake, which prosthesis

you will get, and all of the activities you will still be able to do will help you overcome the unavoidable trauma of surgery.

CONCLUSION

People usually suffer in silence for long periods of time before experiencing burnout. They tend to overestimate their capacities and underestimate their responsibilities. People may bear too heavy a load in their attempts to maintain pride and independence. Caregivers who do so act in good faith, but may not realize that they are exposing themselves and others to harm.

When you feel stress, let people know! No one should ever feel like a failure because they have asked for help. Recognizing that you cannot do it all alone is a strength, not a weakness. With advance preparation, a sense of perspective, and the support of family, friends, and support groups, you can harness the positive potential of stress and avoid burnout.

Chapter 10

Caring for
Your Parents

INTRODUCTION

Children of any age tend to see their parents as caregivers, the ones who are responsible for us and provide us with support, guidance, and advice. As we age, however, these roles change, and are often reversed. Life expectancy continues to increase, and more people are living into their eighties and nineties than ever before. Many super-seniors are active and vibrant, but others face limitations and challenges. These challenges are particularly onerous when they involve physical or psychological disabilities. The number of seniors with disabilities in our society is increasing, and a growing number of children are being forced to decide how best to look after their parents.

Many children, most of whom are now middle-aged, are assuming responsibility for the care of elderly parents. If you make the proper preparations, caring for a parent can strengthen your relationship and make their life better. If you are not prepared for your parents' changing needs, or if you take them into your home without the proper preparations, it can cause problems. This chapter treats the issues and concerns you will have to confront if you are going to help your parents successfully overcome disability, either on their own or in your home.

Owing to government cutbacks in health and social-services spending, as well as increases in institutional costs, there is more pressure than ever for families to absorb the costs of a parent's care. Even if your parents and in-laws are currently healthy and independent, it is important to discuss their wishes in the event of disability. This chapter will help you set your priorities and make informed decisions.

In the last few decades, we have moved away from the practice of caring for parents who can no longer live on their own in the family home. In the nineteenth and early twentieth centuries, the extended family unit was the norm. In the later part of the twentieth century, however, North American society has emphasized personal independence and moved away from this practice. Housing developments designed for the elderly, including retirement communities and nursing homes, have become popular alternatives. In good economic times, pensions and investments enabled many parents to live independently, and the majority of seniors still hope to remain on their own. As seniors grow older, however, they require more physical care, and some become more vulnerable. They need to be in a caring environment where they will be protected, and for an increasing number this environment is the family home.

More and more older citizens are moving into their children's homes. Some, however, require a level of care that can be provided only in an institutional setting. The arrangement that is best for your parents will change over time, and your family will have to adjust to their differing needs. Your parents may move from complete independence to living in your home, then needing an attendant, and finally, requiring institutional care. Providing your parents with care, love, and support will help them maintain their strength and intellectual sharpness. Accurately anticipating the requirements and pressures of care will help maximize your parents' quality of life, and can strengthen your relationship with them.

Grandpa Earl

Michael, an engineer, and Bonita, his wife (who was a nurse by training, but stayed home and took care of their two children), decided to look after Michael's eighty-five-year-old grandfather, Earl, after he became a widower. Earl was a retired history professor, and always had a twinkle in his eye. He frequently took his grandchildren to a local store for candy and ice cream, and told them fascinating bed time stories at night. Earl had a weak heart, however, and in the last two years of his life he was taken to the hospital over thirty times as the result of heart failure.

Although Earl had a history of heart problems before he moved in with his family, the first time he experienced arrhythmia in his new home it was very difficult for the entire family. They called the ambulance, and Earl was hospitalized for a week. The children were very concerned, but their mother assured them that they were capable of handling the situation. Eventually the family came to accept Earl's trips to the hospital as a regular part of life. The ambulance drivers even came to know Earl and the family after several visits.

Michael and Bonita took the requirements of caregiving in stride. They were helped by support from an extended family of fourteen members, each of whom regarded caregiving as shared family responsibility. Some cousins would cook, and others would take care of Earl on weekends when Michael and Bonita wanted to go away. Taking Earl into their home enabled him to live out his final years surrounded by his warm and loving family, and it gave Michael, Bonita, and their children the opportunity to appreciate their wonderful grandpa.

WHAT IS YOUR RESPONSIBILITY TO YOUR PARENT?

These are some basic principles you can follow to fulfil your responsibility to your parents:

- **Help them plan.** If your parents have not prepared for their own disability and/or retirement, it is your responsibility to help them do so. Sit them down and have a frank discussion about living arrangements, medical care, and financial planning with all involved family members. Do this *before* a parent becomes unable to care for himself. Planning in advance will make it easier to negotiate any changes.
- **Consider/respect your parents' wishes.** Like anyone with a disability, your parents should be treated with respect. In planning for your parents' disability, you should consult with them and the other involved relatives, so as to reach a satisfactory decision that maximizes your parents' quality of life. If your parents are no longer able to make viable choices on their own, and have prepared a power of attorney for personal care (see Chapter 13), you may have to make these decisions on their behalf.
- **Focus on quality of life.** Focus your efforts on making your parents' daily living more enjoyable. This may entail providing assistance with everyday tasks your parents may once have taken for granted, including shopping, financial decision-making, recreation, meal preparation, and cleaning.

- **Intervene when appropriate.** If your parents' level of incapacity increases to the point where they may be at risk, you should not be afraid to intercede on their behalf. This may entail providing home care, helping to pay bills, protecting them from con artists, or keeping them involved with your family and the community. Make a genuine commitment to keeping them active. In some communities, you may become legally responsible for your parents' care.

  Parents usually enjoy close interaction with their children, but they may view some of your activities as unwelcome intrusions. Finding the right balance between helping them and respecting their independence requires good judgment.

- **Help locate accommodation.** If your parents can no longer live on their own, you may have to help them find appropriate accommodations. Waiting lists for seniors' residences are often long, and it can take months and even years to get into the best facilities. It takes a lot of legwork to investigate the quality of different facilities, and your parents may require your help in choosing the best one. One of the main accommodation options is taking your parents into your own home.

DECIDING WHERE A PARENT WILL LIVE

In most housing choices prior to institutionalization, parents will be the dominant decision-makers, but you will obviously become more involved if your parent is considering moving into your home. Ideally, a parent's preference should be the deciding factor in where they live, but some seniors' unwillingness to face the reality of their condition makes it necessary for others to become involved in the decision. Individual preference may no longer be the deciding factor, as your family's needs may eclipse what your parent wants. Some people want to continue living on their own when it is no longer possible or safe for them to do so, for example. Others may want to live with children who cannot accommodate them. Try reaching solutions by consensus, to satisfy every family member's needs.

Things to Consider Before Taking Your Parents into Your Home

1. You and your spouse agree, and are committed to your decision.
2. Your children are aware of and involved in your decision.
3. You know exactly what you are undertaking.
4. You know what level of care you are able to provide. This also means that you will recognize the point at which the level of care your parent requires is beyond your capacity to give.
5. If your parent lives in another country or region, you must be sure that you have arranged for any and all necessary medical care. This may involve purchasing insurance or registering for benefits with local government agencies. If you fail to do this, you can run into serious legal and financial difficulties.
6. You have attempted to plan with your parent for any situation that may arise. This may include locating an alternative institutional environment, should one become necessary.

Resolving Differences

Children and parents will not always agree on living arrangements. Conflicts generally arise over four main issues:

1. **They want to live with you, but you are unable to accommodate them.** Most people do not want their parents to reside in a nursing home, but they may not be able to accommodate their needs owing to a lack of space, a financial situation, the level of care needed, or a personality conflict. If it is impossible for you to take your parent into your home, you may wish to contribute to their care in an alternate setting. While rejection may hurt your parents' feelings, you will be doing more harm than good if you bring them into a non-welcoming or inappropriate setting. Be honest and straightforward in telling them why they cannot live with you, but still make the commitment to be as involved as possible in their lives.

2. **They do not want to give up their independence, even if it is for the best.** Sometimes there is little you can do if your parents refuse to consider changing their living arrangements. If your parents are financially independent and strong-willed, they can create a stalemate. Try to overcome the impasse by building a consensus with other members of the family, your parents' friends, physicians, or clergy. A united front may be more effective than if you simply act alone.

   People are sometimes forced to change their living arrangements against their will. Undertake this option only if your parent's health or safety is in danger, and the care that they require cannot be provided elsewhere. In some cases, parents may have to be provided with an ultimatum: "You can no longer care for yourself, and therefore it is necessary for you to hire a caregiver or enter a care facility." This process may be easier if your parents live in rental housing. In some communities, once it is determined that an individual is a danger to himself or others, or is no longer able to provide his own care, the landlord can have him evicted.

3. **You disagree with your spouse over taking responsibility for a parent.** It is usually easier to look after a parent than an in-law. As a result, you might be more favourably disposed to bringing your parents into your home than your spouse is. Because caring for a parent is such an important responsibility, your family must agree before you make this decision. If you cannot convince your spouse that caring for your parent would be a good idea, you may be better off seeking alternate arrangements.

Having your parents move into your home on a trial basis, for a predetermined period, is one possible solution. This test period will give your family the opportunity to see how they adjust to the new living arrangement, and it can help you determine whether you could make it a more permanent situation. If one partner does not give the exercise a real chance, however, then it will not work. Make sure that the ground rules are clear before you start. In particular, your parent should be made aware that the arrangement is not yet permanent, so their expectations are not unduly raised.

4. **You or your spouse reconsider your decision after you have taken a parent into your home.** People seldom realize the amount of work that is involved in providing care for parents. In many instances, a parent's needs increase as they age, and the responsibilities their children encounter become even more onerous. The effort can wear people

down to the point that they feel they can no longer continue providing care. When these feelings emerge, you have a couple of options: you can hire outside caregivers to provide additional care and support, or you can make a change in your living arrangements.

Some parents will realize that things are not working out, and will co-operate in finding an alternate solution. In other cases, parents may be reluctant to leave, and your decision that they should live elsewhere can cause resentment and may damage your relationship. Before you take a parent into your home, discuss the possibility that things may not work out. Hopefully, your parent will agree that if you are not able to provide the level of care he needs, you will look together for alternate arrangements. It is essential that everyone has a complete understanding of the ramifications of your decision before you begin.

WHAT ARE THE ALTERNATIVES?

The housing options for parents are similar to those covered in the chapter on housing. There are, however, some additional factors to take into consideration when making decisions about living accommodations for elderly parents. There are four main modes of housing for senior citizens: independent living, living in a child's home, supported living, and institutionalization.

INDEPENDENT LIVING

Seniors who are living on their own without assistance should be encouraged to maintain this lifestyle. If your parents are independent and are able to take care of themselves, there is no need to rush them into alternate arrangements. Talk to your parents about their needs, and offer assistance if you think it would be appreciated. By visiting frequently you can strengthen your relationship and keep abreast of any needs that may arise. Encourage your parents to live independently for as long as it is reasonably possible.

LOOKING AFTER YOUR PARENTS IN YOUR OWN HOME

Taking a parent into your home can be a very rewarding experience, but it is a decision that should not be taken lightly. Knowing your options will help you decide if this option is right for you.

Where Will They Stay?

Most people are not fortunate enough to own a home with sufficient space for everyone who may wish to live there. Under these circumstances, there are three main options for housing your parents:

1. **A spare room.** If you have a guest room in your home, converting it to a parent's suite is probably the best solution. This will minimize the need for renovations and avoid inconveniencing your family. It will also be more reasonable than residential care or building an addition to your home. If a parent has her own space, it will give her a greater sense of both independence and belonging.

2. **A child's bedroom.** When a grandparent moves in, the lack of space sometimes dictates that one child or more has to relocate and share a room with a sibling. This can be managed smoothly if siblings are willing and able to share space, but older children place a higher value on their independence, and the decreased level of privacy can escalate tensions and lead to conflict.

3. **A "granny suite."** If you have sufficient resources and space, a "granny suite" may be the best solution. A granny suite is a self-contained unit, built as an extension to your home, that serves as a mini-apartment. A typical granny suite contains a bedroom, a washroom, and usually a combination living room/dining room/kitchen. The suite maximizes your parent's independence while keeping him close, so you can ensure his well-being. A granny suite can also be built with an extra bedroom, to accommodate a caregiver. Your parent can even have guests over and not feel that they are imposing on your family.

Many municipal governments encourage the construction of granny suites by offering grants and zoning allowances that would not otherwise be given. Support is often available, and aid can sometimes be found within the community to help with construction. A further benefit is that a granny suite adds to the property value of your home. In the long run, it usually less expensive and more satisfying to build and maintain a granny suite than it is to pay for institutional care.

If You're an Apartment Dweller

In an apartment, space constraints are usually more severe, and rearranging accommodations in a small apartment may create many difficulties. There is usually no room to expand, unless you move to another apartment. An option that is becoming more popular is renting (or having your parents rent) a suite in the same building. This has a similar effect as building a granny suite and avoids the stresses of living in the same space.

Benefits to Bringing Parents into Your Home

- **A closer family unit.** A grandparent living in the family home can re-establish or strengthen family bonds. It increases a grandparent's sense of belonging and importance, and allows for more frequent expressions of love and affection. This feeling of belonging helps maintain self-esteem and increases the motivation to stay active. The vibrancy of more youthful family members stimulates grandparents and provides a welcome contrast to a solitary lifestyle, which can be lonely and isolated. Your children will also gain a greater appreciation for their grandparent.

- **Help around the home.** Many grandparents provide useful support for their families by caring for children and helping with light household tasks. Most parents who live with their children want to contribute to the household, and are willing to assume some responsibilities. As co-residents, grandparents have an added stake in keeping their home clean, growing a beautiful garden, making enjoyable meals, or performing other roles. Some parents may be reluctant to perform these tasks, however, as they may not want to intrude on your domain. Go out of your way to make sure that they are involved in the family home. Even a small contribution can help make your life easier.

- **Help with family expenses.** Frequently, parents are in a position to contribute to family expenses. Because they no longer have to pay rent or a mortgage, parents may have the resources available to pay for their own needs in your home, and perhaps contribute a little something extra. Some parents have contributed to their children's mortgages in order to express their appreciation and their feeling of inclusion as a member of the household.

Problems with Bringing Parents into the Family Home

Although there are many benefits to taking a parent into the home, you should carefully consider the problems that sometimes occur. When you're taking on this responsibility, the tasks involved usually appear to be relatively simple. But as your parents age, it becomes more challenging to provide for their physical, psychological, and social needs.

- **Changes to family dynamics.** Just as a new baby changes the household, so does the addition of an older individual. Family members will experience a loss of privacy. There is always one more person at the dinner table, one more person to be included in family activities, and one more person to squabble over the remote control. Many grandparents have different moral standards than their grandchildren, and some teenagers will find that they do not share all of their grandparents' values. Personality differences may also cause significant family problems. These problems can be averted if household roles and rules are discussed as soon as the grandparent moves in. Any other conflicts that arise should be openly discussed and resolved as quickly as possible.
- **Interference with social activities.** Grandparents often have different standards and expectations than you or your children. They may have very different tastes in music, TV, and movies; they may want the house to be quiet early; and they may expect a different level of behaviour than you and your children are accustomed to. When you go out, they will sometimes expect to be brought along, and will sometimes want to be brought home early when the entire family goes out. A friend of mine who took care

of his mother used to tell me that this ninety-year-old woman waited up for him every night!

When grandparents' physical and mental faculties deteriorate, it can create awkward situations for you and your children. Parents may make inconsiderate requests. They may place heavy demands on your time, and be very inflexible about when guests can visit and when they should leave. They may also be very demanding about the time they want to spend with *their* friends. These situations can raise the anxiety levels of all family members.

- **Increased costs.** Sometimes, taking a parent into your home can be expensive. Because of a parent's deteriorating eyesight, hearing, or motor skills, it is often necessary to retrofit your home with safety bars, special lighting, wider doorways, and other renovations. These accommodations can cost thousands of dollars.

  You may have to hire personnel on a full- or part-time basis to care for a parent when you are away from home. Some individuals must be closely supervised, especially older people who smoke on a regular basis. Lapses in attention on the part of elderly smokers are a major cause of household and institutional fires. Prescription drugs, special diets, therapies, and assistive technologies can all be very expensive, and are often your responsibility.

SUPPORTED LIVING

An option favoured by many seniors and their children is independent living with outside support. This means that your parents live in their own home or apartment with the assistance of personnel who perform a number of duties. These people carry out tasks that your parents find difficult or impossible to do on their own, thereby allowing them to maintain their independence. They are able to live in relative freedom as long as help is available.

Family members sometimes assume this responsibility, but caregivers are usually either professionals or volunteers who provide a variety of in-home services. They are trained to recognize any medical crisis, and they know how to respond or who to contact in an emergency. The services provided by caregivers can include:

- medical supervision;
- nursing care;
- managing finances;
- physical and occupational therapy;
- housekeeping;
- shopping;
- meal preparation;
- bathing and toileting;
- administering drugs;
- providing transportation;
- social and recreational activities.

Determine with your parents which tasks they require help with and which they can still do on their own. The object of supported living is to maintain as much of their independence as possible.

Independent Living with Full-Time Supervision

Sometimes even those with the most severe disabilities want to continue to live on their own. This may be possible, but only with twenty-four-hour supervision and care. The main benefit of this strategy is that it establishes and maintains a constant level of interaction between the patient and her caregiver. The main drawback is that it is a very expensive option.

Financial Support for Independent Living

Full-time care can cost between $2,500 and $10,000 a month, and sometimes more. Personnel, medication, and housing expenses constitute the bulk of the costs. In some cases, there is government support for such care, and service clubs occasionally also offer aid. This is important, because most people's insurance and savings are not sufficient to meet these requirements, especially if attendant care is needed for more than a couple of months. Whether your parent will benefit from this kind of care may depend on your financial circumstances. In most situations, an institution is a more viable alternative for people with severe disabilities than twenty-four-hour-a-day, in-home care.

Supported Living Communities (SLCs)

SLCs are protected and secure environments that are specifically designed to meet the needs of the elderly. Most SLCs are apartment complexes reserved for elderly residents. In these surroundings an individual lives on his own with the support of caregiving staff who are on call twenty-four hours a day to provide assistance in case of emergencies. Staff members check on the residents on a regular basis to ensure their well-being and to help administer medication. The staff also help with housecleaning and meal preparation, and organize activities for the residents. Many seniors benefit from the combination of independence with increased support, and enjoy the companionship of people who have similar needs and concerns.

The Benefits of Supported Living

- **Greater independence.** In SLCs, seniors do not have to conform to institutional rules or standards. They maintain control over meal planning, recreational and social choices, and bedtimes. Residents make the vast majority of their own decisions in supported living communities.

- **Individualized care.** The residents' care is tailored to their individual needs, not determined by a generic blueprint dictated by institutional policy. Individualized care provides greater opportunities for personal relationships to develop between people with disabilities and their caregivers.
- **Maximized activity.** The independence and stimulation provided in SLCs motivates people to remain active. Because they are still responsible for many tasks, people in supported living environments are usually more energetic than their counterparts in institutions.
- **Self-esteem and dignity.** Residents in SLCs do not feel dependent on outsiders for their well-being. Their responsibilities within the SLC enhance their self-respect. Service is looked on as a supplement to residents' abilities, not something that renders them dependent.

Drawbacks to Supported Living Communities

- **Cost.** The main drawback to supported living is cost. Chapters 11, 12, and 13 detail the strategies that will help you to overcome monetary limitations through the use of support groups, charities, investments, and planning for disability.
- **Exposure to strangers.** Because caregivers perform highly intimate tasks, recipients of care may be embarrassed and would prefer to be looked after by family members. It takes time for anyone to become accustomed to a new caregiver, but a trusting relationship can eventually be built.
- **Problems with personnel.** The vast majority of caregivers are committed, honest, and reliable. Some caregivers, however, do not fulfil their responsibilities. They may not

show up reliably for work, or may perform at an unsatisfactory level. Some caregivers have stolen from their elderly patients, and some patients have even been abused. Care and vigilance in selecting and supervising personnel can avert these problems.

INSTITUTIONAL LIVING

We discussed the positives and negatives of institutional living in Chapter 3, and they are the same for seniors as for anyone else with a disability. The two main forms of institutional living for seniors are residences that cater to people with specific disabilities and nursing homes, which provide high-level care for seniors with extensive disabilities.

There are several keys to making a parent's experience in a nursing home as positive as possible. These strategies are elaborated on in greater detail in the chapter on housing.

- **Cost does not guarantee quality.** Even the most expensive homes may not provide reliable and regular care. It is often a good idea to hire a part-time attendant to look after your parent's personal needs when you are unable to visit. Elderly people benefit from continuous interaction; if they are left in an isolated situation, their condition can deteriorate.
- **Be involved.** Make sure that your parent is not "warehoused." If the nursing home knows that you are actively involved in your parent's care, they will almost always be more attentive to her needs. Visit as often as possible, and encourage other family members, friends, and clergy to visit — anyone who can make her life more interesting. Consult with the staff so you are constantly up to date on your parent's status.

- **Help them stay active.** Take your parent out of the residence as often as possible. Encourage him to be involved with the facility's activities. A high level of activity has been proven to increase the quality of life of the elderly, and to help maintain their physical and mental health.

Alice

Sally and Ted lived in Boston. They had four children, ages seven through nineteen. When Sally's father died, her mother, Alice, decided to come and live with her family for a short period of time, as she did not want to stay in the large home she had shared with her husband for over forty years. Alice planned to stay with her daughter until she could sell her home and decide where she wanted to live. During the first week that Alice lived with her daughter, she slipped on the ice in front of the home and broke her knee in three places. After two weeks in the hospital she moved back in with Sally and Ted. Her mobility was severely restricted, and she was unable to contemplate looking for a new residence.

Alice learned to walk again with a cane, but she remained in discomfort. She also decided not to look for other accommodations at all. Whenever Alice was home alone she became very disconcerted. When Sally and Ted would leave the house, Alice would tell them that she did not like being abandoned. Over a period of several months, Alice's demands increased. Her criticisms and accusations led to numerous arguments and shouting matches.

Sally and Ted were working hard to pay off their mortgage and take care of their children. They loved Alice dearly, but were finding it increasingly difficult to maintain the necessary level of care.

One major point of contention was the decision to take a family ski holiday over the Christmas vacation without Alice. After much haggling they convinced her to stay in a seniors' residence for six days while they were away. The family returned rested and relaxed, and once again prepared to deal with the ongoing difficulties of living with their grandmother.

To their surprise, when they returned home Alice insisted on remaining at the seniors' residence. She had enjoyed having all of the other people around, and taking part in the wide range of activities that were offered. The home had a pool, and a physical and occupational therapy program. Staff organized frequent outings to plays, movies, concerts, and bingo. She told her family that there was "never a dull moment" at the home, where she had met a number of new friends. She was determined to stay.

Although the nursing home cost $2,000 a month more than living with her children did, Sally was able to convince her three brothers to share their mother's residential costs. In this instance, Alice was well suited to the residential environment. She needed stimulation and therapy that could not be provided at home, where people were busy at work or at school and did not always have enough time to spend with her. Alice realized that she was happiest in the residential setting.

Deciding on Institutionalization

An individual will rarely express the need to move to a more restrictive setting on their own. If you are concerned about your parent's health or safety, you should discuss your feelings with your parent, other family members, a physician, and a representative of local family or social services. Staff at a supported living centre can also initiate action if they feel that they can no longer provide adequate care.

After the process has been initiated, the first step is a review by social services, which includes the input of members of the family and the family physician. When it is determined that an individual's needs can be met only in a nursing home environment, the social-service worker will search for an appropriate facility and recommend the individual for the placement.

It is often extremely difficult to find a nursing-home bed, and seniors can be forced to wait for more than a year. In the meantime, people with severe health problems may be housed in hospitals or in their children's homes. If you feel that your parents may eventually need the care of a nursing home, it is advisable to start the process early. By placing their names on a waiting list as soon as possible, any delay can be minimized. Even if they are at the top of the list, they may still be pushed back by emergency cases who have an immediate need for the care.

Concerns over Entering an Institution

Try to anticipate your parents' needs. Be aware of the residential options and the time needed to arrange this type of care. Some individuals get help from local social-service agencies, which are aware of the facilities that provide the best available care. Discuss the quality of care, level of programming, recreational opportunities, and available resources with your parents before any decision is made.

CONCLUSION

Hopefully, your parents will be able to maintain their independence for as long as possible. Even so, you should discuss your parents' living options in advance so that you will not have to make important decisions in a vacuum should a crisis occur. Making an important decision on the spur of the moment can lead to all sorts of avoidable difficulties. Taking the time to lay the groundwork for your decision will improve your chances for success. Bringing parents or in-laws into your home can be very rewarding for you and your family when everyone is involved and supportive.

PART 3

Protecting

Your Future

Chapter
11

The Importance of a Protection Plan

INTRODUCTION

Despite my many years of experience in the field of disability as an activist and an educator, I, like too many others, was completely unprepared when I had my heart attack. I wasn't ready for all of the changes I had to make, but I was fortunate to have a safety net that allowed me some time to adjust. The long-term disability coverage provided by my university would have guaranteed my income until age sixty-five, at which point I would have qualified for full retirement benefits. In addition, I had full medical coverage. My only out-of-pocket expense was for TV rental. If I had been forced to pay for the full cost of my care (surgery, medication, rehabilitation, etc.), it would have been more than $300,000. And if I had not had excellent disability insurance, we would have been forced to declare bankruptcy and we would have lost our home, our cars, our retirement savings — everything.

217

Despite all of my problems, I was lucky. Because I had both medical and disability coverage, my family was protected from suffering financial trauma on top of the emotional trauma. Many others are not so fortunate. One of my co-patients in the cardiac ward, a construction worker in his late thirties, told me that his heart attack was probably going to bring on the financial ruin of his family. Although he had comprehensive medical coverage, he had no long-term disability insurance. His wife had never worked, and her efforts were not going to be able to make up for his lost income. He foresaw that he was going to be unable to meet his mortgage payments, his car payments, and his credit-card debts. He could never go back to work at his old job in heavy labour. He said, "Within a few months, my wife and I will probably be forced to sell our house, our two cars, and we may declare bankruptcy or even go on welfare."

Stories like this are all too common. People are unaware of the dangers they face, and many wrongly assume they are protected. Most people do not know what they would need to survive such a crisis. By sharing with you what I have learned, I hope to show you how to prepare yourself in the event that a disability occurs to you or to someone you love. If you prepare yourself to deal with disability — emotionally and financially — you will be able to overcome almost any challenge.

If you are just embarking on your working career, what would you guess your chances are of encountering, before you reach sixty-five, a disability that prevents you from working for at least ninety days? Ten percent? Twenty percent? Maybe 33 percent, a one in three chance? Wrong! If you are a twenty-five-year-old, your chances of suffering a disability that prevents you from working for at least three months is *58 percent!*

Most people don't want to think about disability. They feel it is a remote possibility that they don't have to consider. They

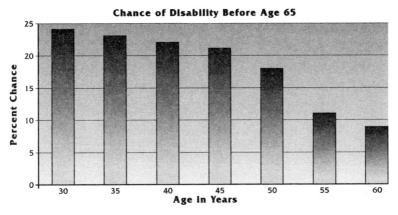

Chance of Disability Before Age 65

could not be more wrong! Statistics show that the risk of disability is real. If you happen to be one of the 58 percent who experience a serious disability before the age of sixty-five — say, at the age of forty — how long, on average, do you think the disability would last? Five months? Ten months? Eighteen months? The average duration of disability at the age of forty is 3.1 years, or thirty-seven months! This is a time when it will be difficult, if not impossible, to work. Costs will mount, and if you are not protected, you and your family could face financial ruin.

The ability to earn income is your most important financial asset. This asset, however, is dependent on your health. It can be

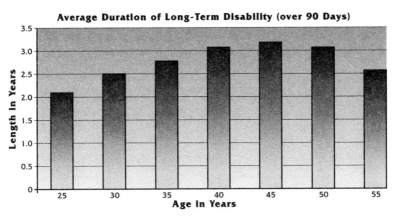

Average Duration of Long-Term Disability (over 90 Days)

taken away by disability, just when you need it the most. The costs of disability can be staggering, running into the hundreds of thousands of dollars. It is important not only that you are able to pay for the costs of disability, but also that you can maintain your family's standard of living and protect your home, your investments, and your retirement savings.

Because of the dangers disability can pose if you are unprepared, it is vital to make provisions to mitigate against the impact. This chapter will introduce you to the basic principles and building blocks with which you can protect yourself and your family. The next chapter will explain each of these options in detail, and describe what you should look for, what you should avoid, guidelines on how much you should spend and who you should consult. We will also discuss the legal-planning measures you can undertake to ensure that your family is protected in the event that you experience disability.

IT CAN'T HAPPEN TO ME

Until they look at the figures, most people feel that they have a slim or non-existent chance of suffering a disability. As a result, the majority of people are not even aware of the kinds of insurance available. If they are aware, many feel that it is an unneeded expense. When you are starting a career or beginning a family, the thought that it could all end suddenly is the last thing on your mind. Many people who have reached middle age are similarly unprotected, having allowed their policies to lapse or having declined disability insurance altogether. Many people prefer to use their disposable income for housing, other investments, or recreation. In addition, thousands of people who have a disability-insurance plan at work simply assume that they are adequately covered, when in fact their policies are often substandard. As a result, more than half the population lacks adequate protection against disability. Most people feel that insurance is a poor buy until they need it. By then it is too late.

Contrary to popular opinion, you have a far greater chance of suffering a disability at an early age than you do of dying young. Furthermore, disability is more frequently caused by illness than by accident.

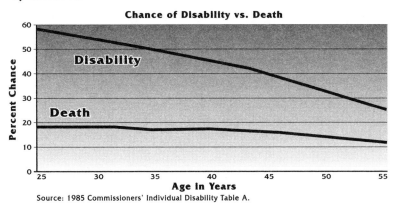

Chance of Disability vs. Death

Source: 1985 Commissioners' Individual Disability Table A.

THE IMPORTANCE OF FINANCIAL PLANNING FOR DISABILITY

Many people have a financial plan, but the majority have not built in provisions for disability. Your whole financial portfolio can go down the tubes, however, if all of your revenues have to be redirected to pay the costs of disability. During a period of disability, a financial plan established while you are healthy may be the only thing that can save you from disaster. Incorporating the appropriate insurance into your portfolio will ensure that your other investments will not have to be liquidated to pay your expenses during this time of uncertainty. Provisions can be made to ensure that your financial circumstances will not be altered by disability on a day-to-day basis or over the long term. If you plan properly, you will be able to build and protect the nest egg you are putting away for your children's education and your retirement.

Our focus when discussing financial planning is not on saving for retirement, playing the stock market, knowing how to purchase the right mutual funds, or learning how to make money by following demographic trends. There are excellent financial-planning guides on the market that focus on these areas, and many of them are listed in the back of this book. Our focus is on building a stable financial strategy that will protect your income, assets, and investments in the case of disability. Once you have built in the proper protections, you will be able to move on and expand your financial portfolio into other areas.

Any bona fide financial plan requires a solid foundation. Protection from disability is just one element, but without it all of your other investments may collapse. If you guarantee the sustainability of your assets and the continuation of your income, you will be able to pursue more diverse investments — secure in the knowledge that even in the worst-case scenario, your family's finances are fundamentally sound.

The Costs of Disability

If you are not covered by an adequate medical plan, the initial costs of disability can be astronomical. Double-bypass surgery, in many jurisdictions, can cost $300,000. One day in the cardiac ward can cost upward of $1,200. Even if your basic care is covered, cutbacks to the health system mean that the personal care you receive from hospital staff may be insufficient. Many hospitals now recommend that you hire outside assistance if your family or friends are unable to provide care. Ordinary attendant care (people to perform light housekeeping, shop, provide meals) starts at approximately ten dollars an hour. Private nursing, which may be desirable or even necessary following surgery, can cost more than $200 for an eight-hour shift. Full-time, twenty-four-hour nursing can cost more than $4,000 a week.

The costs for rehabilitation can also be astronomical. Occupational therapists, physiotherapists, speech pathologists, and other similar paramedical personnel usually charge $50 to $125 an hour. Psychiatrists' and psychologists' rates vary widely. Subsidized counselling is available for free, or for a minimal charge. Private fees, however, can cost $100 dollars an hour or more. Specialized clinics, which teach people how to use wheelchairs and manipulate artificial limbs, can sometimes cost in excess of $10,000 a month. Specialized cancer clinics and other treatment facilities are similarly expensive.

Prescription drug costs can vary from ten to several hundred dollars a week, and few health plans cover alternative therapies, which are growing in popularity. Bills from chiropractors, homeopaths, acupuncturists, and pain-management therapists can all be expensive. In-home caregivers charge rates similar to those of hospital staff, and long-term institutional care can cost between $5,000 and $10,000 a month. Specialized or highly intensive care, including MRIs, CAT scans, large numbers of x-rays, transplants, and cutting-edge prosthetics, may not be covered by your health plan. These services can be prohibitively expensive.

If you experience a permanent disability, there will be further long-term costs, including specialized transportation, retrofitting your residence or moving to a more accessible home, job retraining, specialized equipment, ongoing prescriptions, specialized clothing, and specialized recreation. With a degenerative condition such as multiple sclerosis or lupus, which gets worse over time, the costs continue to rise. All of these necessary items are above and beyond your everyday expenses, such as a mortgage, rent, utilities, other insurance, taxes, food, clothing, transportation, and recreation.

Loss of Income

It is possible that you could bear some or all of the costs of a serious disability if you were able to keep working full time, but many people who experience disability are unable to work for at least ninety days — and the average length of disability is more than two years. If you are off work for an extended period of time, numerous pressures can start to build:

- If you are completely unable to work, you may lose your job as a result of your disability.
- It may become difficult to pay the costs of your debts; banks and other financial institutions are also more likely to call in loans.
- While you are unable to work, you may not be able to find someone who can effectively take over the operation of your business; if you are forced to sell your business, it may be difficult to get fair value for your assets.
- It may become increasingly difficult to continue saving for your retirement, your children's education, or a vacation.
- If you are on a fixed income, your level of disposable income will steadily decrease, due to inflation.

Francine

A fifty-seven-year-old woman named Francine was seriously injured in a car accident caused by a drunk driver. She was hospitalized for nine months, during which time she underwent five surgeries. Following her hospitalization, she had seven more surgeries, which attempted to relieve her almost constant pain. The driver, who had assets valued at less than $10,000, was uninsured. Fortunately, Francine had a $2-million car-insurance policy that was able to cover her costs. She had purchased optional underinsurance protection, which allowed her to sue her own car-insurance company for the damage she sustained in the accident. If she had not purchased this coverage, she would have had only minimal coverage for her devastating injuries.

Francine underwent an economic and health assessment to determine the immediate and long-term costs of her care. Assessors are independent professionals contracted by a victim's lawyer to provide an accurate projection of the costs on which a disability claim can be based. The assessors evaluated Francine's needs in a wide variety of areas: medical, non-medical, mobility, personal care, personal support services, professional services, residential, home maintenance, and recreation. The final breakdown of costs considered almost ninety different items, ranging from drug prescriptions (which cost $620 per year), to a scooter, wheelchair, and other mobility aids (which cost $2,050 per year), to homemaking and household cleaning services (which cost $7,050 per year). The estimated cost of Francine's care over a five-year period was $195,000. Her life expectancy is another twenty-five years, and the potential cost of care over that time could exceed $1 million. If you were in an accident of a similar magnitude, could you pay these costs?

How Can I Pay the Costs of My Disability?

After disability strikes, there are several ways you can pay your living expenses, mortgage or rent, utilities, clothing, and taxes:

1. **Liquidate savings.** It is sometimes possible to take money you have set aside for other purposes (retirement plans, educational plans, bank accounts) and direct it towards meeting your costs. However, if you saved 5 percent of your income each year, just six months of disability could wipe out ten years of savings. Unless you are a multi-millionaire, you will not be able to sustain your standard of

living following a long-term disability on savings alone.

2. **Borrow.** Banks have always been hesitant to lend money to people with disabilities, because they are viewed as poor credit risks. If your disability prevents you from working, getting a new loan will be almost impossible. Even if you have a good relationship with your bank manager, it is unlikely that you will be able to secure a loan if you have no viable source of income. When people first experience disability, they also have a tendency to run up serious debts on their credit cards. Because of the high rate of interest on most cards, this can compound your credit crunch and lead to an unsustainable debt burden.

   Some people also borrow from family or friends to try to meet the costs of their disabilities. Loved ones may be less stringent than banks when lending money, but if you have difficulty paying off your loans, you risk straining or even losing these relationships. Unless it is absolutely necessary, avoid borrowing from friends or family.

3. **Use your spouse's income.** If you are your family's principal breadwinner and are unable to work because of a disability, your family's income will be significantly reduced. Determine if your remaining household income will be sufficient to pay for all household bills, as well as the additional expenses you will encounter. In most instances, the secondary earner's income is factored into the household budget, not viewed as surplus. As a result, most families cannot rely on only one income to sustain them in times of disability.

4. **Liquidate assets.** Some people are forced to sell their possessions and property in order to pay the costs of disability. Cars, jewellery, furniture, homes, and other valuable possessions have all been sold by individuals desperate for

funds. Selling all of your most valuable possessions can diminish your quality of life, however. Furthermore, when you are forced to liquidate your most valuable possessions, it can be difficult to get a fair market price. Some people will try to take advantage of you if they sense that you are desperate.

5. **Apply for government assistance.** Government funding is sometimes available from municipal, state, or provincial sources. Safety nets such as welfare, disability benefits, and workers' compensation can provide some funding, but these benefits are usually for a fixed period of time and are capped at a far lower level than most incomes. The average benefit from government programs will amount to only 66 percent of the poverty level. If it is possible, take advantage of government assistance, but do not rely on it to meet all of your needs.

6. **Purchase an individually tailored disability plan.** An individually tailored disability plan avoids many of the problems associated with your other options. Your plan may include disability insurance, life insurance, critical-care illness insurance, business insurance, and other forms of supplementary coverage. This is the best option you can choose to protect yourself from disability.

WHY A DISABILITY PLAN IS THE BEST OPTION

Because the costs of disability can run into the hundreds of thousands of dollars in a very short period of time, it is important to establish a guaranteed source of income that will be sufficient to meet your family's needs. A disability plan can be engineered to fit your particular circumstances and your budget. If you have a disability plan, you will not have to resort to other, less effective strategies.

The Components of a Disability Plan

Disability Insurance

Disability insurance can protect your income while you are affected by disability. Disability insurance will provide you with a certain percentage of your original income (usually 60–70 percent), and it can be designed to cover the additional costs of your disability. The level of benefits, exclusions, taxability, and length of coverage varies from plan to plan.

Life Insurance

If you don't have life insurance before you experience a disability, it is usually impossible to purchase after. Also, if you have a sibling or parent who dies young or is affected by a chronic illness, the cost of your coverage may increase substantially. Some companies may even deny you a policy. The best option is to purchase a small life-insurance policy early in your working career, preferably one that includes a provision allowing you to increase your level of coverage at any time at pre-defined rates. Some life-insurance policies build up a cash value that can also be used as an emergency fund during a time of disability to pay for your cost of care or to service debts.

Critical Care/Critical Illness Insurance

This form of insurance provides a lump-sum payment that is designed to help financially at the onset of a critical illness. If you survive for a specified length of time after diagnosis (usually thirty days), the company will provide a large, one-time payoff that can help you to meet all of your expenses and avert any potential threats to your lifestyle. The conditions covered by this form of insurance must be specified in the plan, and payments are based on health only. If you suffer a disability owing to a condition specified on your contract, you get paid, end of story.

Business Insurance

Specialized coverage can be purchased to protect businesses in the event of a disability that prevents the owner from working. The insurance can cover overhead costs, payroll, and the loss of a key employee. It can also be designed to ensure that you get a fair price in the event that your disability forces you to sell your business. This form of protection is particularly vital for doctors, dentists, hairdressers, tradesmen, and any other professionals and businesspeople who have to rely on their physical skills.

Supplementary Coverage

Many people have partial or limited disability insurance through their place of employment. This coverage, however, is usually insufficient to completely protect an individual from the impact of disability. Benefits are taxable and tend to be lower, the benefit period may be capped, and you may be forced to return to work against your will. Supplementary coverage allows you to "top up" these benefits to ensure that you have a comprehensive plan.

Other Forms of Insurance

Automobile insurance, mortgage insurance, investment insurance, and other forms of coverage are other possible components of a protection plan.

CONCLUSION

Insurance plans can be grouped into three main categories: "Cadillac plans," average plans, and minimal plans. A Cadillac plan offers a "liberal" definition of disability, and will provide the best available protection until you turn sixty-five. It will contain all or a vast majority of the options described above. A Cadillac plan will cover you in all financial eventualities.

Average plans provide middle-range protection. Benefit levels will be lower than in a Cadillac plan, and you are seldom insured to sixty-five. Some of these plans have strict time limits on benefits, and they will rarely include inflation riders, coverage for experimental therapies, or other additional features. Someone with this type of plan may be forced to assume an alternate form of employment if he is unable to resume his original career. These plans will provide solid short-term protection, but they cannot always be counted on to provide lifelong support for disability.

Minimal plans will provide coverage for a maximum of two years, and if the disability is not total, they may not pay at all. These plans will not pay a high level of benefits, they will not pay for experimental therapies, and they will not cover the entire spectrum of disabling conditions, such as carpal tunnel syndrome or chronic back pain. Most people just assume that their long-term disability insurance covers everything, but this is rarely the case. The majority of employers purchase average or minimal plans, as Cadillac coverage is very expensive. Make sure that the plan you choose is suited to your needs and provides appropriate protection.

By carefully researching your options and working with the appropriate personnel, you can devise a plan that protects you and your family. In Chapter 12, we illustrate how you can build a comprehensive protection plan.

Chapter 12

How to Build a Protection Plan

INTRODUCTION

In the previous chapter, we explained the risks you face and why a disability plan that takes all of these factors into account is your best option. In this chapter, we will go into more detail on how to make sure that you get the legal and financial coverage that is right for your family. What constitutes the "right" insurance plan will vary from person to person, and depends on age, income, family size, debts, and a host of other factors, but there are some basic procedures that everyone should follow when building a comprehensive protection package.

To ensure that you make the best decision, consult with a range of professionals, including financial planners, insurance agents, lawyers (preferably an insurance specialist), accountants, and bank managers. After you experience a disability, you may also require the services of an insurance assessor, who will usually be affiliated with your lawyer. This chapter explains the different types of insurance in greater detail, and describes how an effective protection plan can be built.

THE COMPONENTS OF A PROTECTION PLAN

Disability Insurance

A disability insurance contract will make sure that your income is replaced during a time of sickness or injury. Not all disability insurance contracts are the same, and you should take your time exploring the range of options available before you make your decision. The most important feature in a disability contract is the definition of disability. You should try to purchase a contract with the most liberal definition possible.

The Different Definitions of Disability

1. **Own occupation.** Under this definition, you are considered to be disabled if you are unable to perform the substantial and material duties of your own occupation, regardless of your ability to engage in another occupation. This is the most comprehensive definition available in a disability contract. It pays benefits while still allowing you to work at another job. Some "own occupation" policies, however, require you to deduct any additional income you earn from your benefits. Each policy can be different!

   Even though it is the most comprehensive form of coverage, you still have to be careful. Within some occupations, there is a vast difference in jobs and physical requirements for the job. For example, a surgeon may not want to be forced back to work as a medical researcher.

Brent

Brent, a chiropractor making $75,000 a year, developed arthritis in his hands and was unable to run his practice any longer. As soon as his claim was verified, the insurance company began paying benefits, at 70 percent of his original salary. Although he could have retired on the benefits from his insurance contract, Brent was given the opportunity to teach at a local chiropractic college, at a salary of $52,000 per year. Even though he earns a second income that approaches that of his original practice, Brent still receives full disability benefits, because he is unable to perform the duties of his "own occupation." Brent was not forced back to work, but chose to pick up a secondary occupation. As a result, his income after the disability actually increased to $104,500 dollars a year. Although Brent obviously missed being able to practise, the right disability coverage turned a potential disaster into a positive situation. If you want to be able to choose if and where you work following a serious disability, this is the best option available.

2. **Any occupation.** If you are interested in guaranteeing your income, and are not as concerned about the possibility of switching professions, then this is a suitable option. This type of coverage insures your ability to work generally, not your ability to work at your current profession. You will be fully covered if you are unable to perform any occupation for which you are reasonably qualified by education, training, or experience. However, if you are unable to perform the day-to-day duties of your job, but can still be retrained or rehabilitated to perform another job of any kind, *then the policy will not pay.* You may be forced into another occupation, even if there is no job available or you no longer wish to continue working. This

policy rarely pays through to age sixty-five, and sometimes it never pays at all!

Dennis

Dennis is a thirty-eight-year-old steelworker who injured his back carrying steel coils. He was unable to work at all for six months, during which time he was fully covered by his "any occupation" disability policy. After intensive rehabilitation, Dennis's health improved significantly. He was still unable to perform the heavy lifting that would have allowed him to resume his old job, but he was rehabilitated to the point where he was able to take an office job with the same company. As soon as he was healthy enough to return to work, his benefits were cut off and he was forced to begin his new job. Fortunately, Dennis earned the same salary at his new job as he had in his previous position.

3. **Regular occupation.** This is the most common version of individually purchased disability contracts. It is what most people who are self-employed, professionals, or on contract will purchase. "Regular occupation" contracts offer a very liberal definition of disability and will pay out for one of three reasons:

- if you cannot perform the important duties of your job, and you are not engaged in any other occupation;
- if you experience an earned-income loss of 75 percent or more;
- if you do not experience an income loss of 75 percent or more, but you have been classified as unable to work due to disability.

Bill

Bill is the owner of a shipping company that employs sixty-five people. He contracted prostate cancer and was unable to work for an extended period of time. Another individual was brought in to conduct the day-to-day activities of the operation while Bill was gone, and the revenues of his company did not change over the short term. Because Bill's contract was tied to the performance of the company, he continued to draw his salary. In addition, the insurance company paid him 67 percent of his original salary, because he was unable to perform the key duties of his occupation.

4. **Twenty-four-month regular occupation, changing to any occupation after twenty-four months.** This definition is very common among group plans offered by employers. Under this definition, the disability contract will pay if the insured individual is unable to perform the duties of his own occupation in the first twenty-four months of a disability. Even if you can perform another job, you are not required to work.

After twenty-four months, if the insured individual cannot perform any occupation for which he is reasonably qualified by education, training, or experience, then the contract will still pay, until he reaches the age of sixty-five. If the person insured is deemed able to work at another position for any employer, the insurance company will send a letter listing the range of alternative occupations available. The individual who has experienced the disability will then be forced to choose one of the work options or face a total loss of income, even if there is no job available.

Note: "Any occupation" and "twenty-four-month regular

occupation" are most commonly found in disability contracts offered by employers. The premiums for these are cheaper than "own occupation" and "regular occupation."

Other Important Features

There are several optional features in disability contracts that you should consider.

Partial Disability

This option will provide benefits if a disability prevents you from carrying out your full workload. You do not have to be totally disabled. If you experience an earned income loss of between 20 and 75 percent, then a portion of your disability benefit will be paid.

For example, a chronic back problem prevents Shirley from working full days as a computer programmer. Because she is able to work only four hours a day, or half of her regular shift, she is paid 50 percent of her disability benefit every month. Shirley underwent intensive therapy for her back, which enabled her to increase her workload to six hours a day. Thereafter she received 25 percent of her disability benefit.

Measures to Guarantee Contract Security

The premiums for individually purchased disability contracts are based on the age of the person insured when the contract is purchased. Therefore, the younger you are, the lower the premium. When you purchase your policy, make sure that the premiums cannot be altered. Also, look for a policy that is "non-cancellable and guaranteed renewable," meaning that the contract's wording cannot be changed once it has been issued. With this provision, the insurance company cannot cancel the policy, even if your health changes over the life of the contract.

Inflation

No one can live on a fixed income for his entire life, because the cost of living is always increasing. You should look for a disability contract that adjusts for inflation. If at all possible, a compounding inflation factor is preferable to simple interest.

For example, if an individual with a salary of $60,000 per year goes on disability insurance, a policy with a standard benefit of 60 percent of earned income would pay him $36,000 per year. If the policy is not indexed for inflation, however, its real value could diminish significantly over time. At a rate of inflation of 2 percent, the value of the policy would decrease to $32,446 in real dollars after five years. After ten years, the policy's real value would be only $29,351. If the rate of inflation increased to 5 percent, the same policy would be worth only $27,995 in real dollars after five years. After ten years, the real value of the benefits will have decreased to $21,663. That is less than 60 percent of the policy's original value. A decrease of this magnitude in your purchasing power can seriously harm your quality of life.

Future Insurability Options

This feature gives you the opportunity to purchase additional, future benefits when your pre-disability income goes up. With a future insurability option, the insurance company will allow you to make this purchase regardless of your health.

For example, a medical doctor purchased a disability policy while still a resident. She was not making a substantial income, and was therefore unable to purchase a large benefit. Five years later, her income had increased substantially, and she applied to increase her benefit level. But in the intervening five years, she had developed a problem with hypertension, and she was worried that she would be forced to pay an extra premium or might even be denied the increase in benefit. Despite her health problems, though, she was able to purchase the increased benefit without a drastic increase in her premium, thanks to the future insurability option in her contract.

Return of Premium
Some insurance companies reward the policyholder for remaining disability-free. If, after a period of eight to ten years, an insured individual has not made a claim on her disability insurance, or if she has made only a very small claim, the insurance company will reward her by refunding up to 75 percent of all premiums paid. This provision makes many people think twice about submitting a claim on a disability that is not serious. It also puts the person who is insured in a win-win situation. If you experience a disability, you get paid; if you do not experience disability, you still get paid.

Underwriting
It is very important to purchase a policy that will confirm and approve your health status when you apply. This process is known as underwriting. Underwriting prevents an insurer from being able to avoid paying your claim. A contract that is issued automatically but is not underwritten until the claim is submitted (which could be many years later) can be very dangerous. You must disclose any and all information about your health and income when you sign the policy. The payment of a claim can be delayed, contested, or even denied if you have not provided all of the relevant information, even if the omission was accidental.

Waiver of Premium

It is wise to invest in this option if you have other insurance policies and investments. This feature ensures that all of your
premiums will continue to be paid during a time of disability. As
most disability contracts insure only 60 to 67 percent of your
earned income, your "take home" income may be significantly
less than it was while you were working. When it comes to a
choice between paying for your mortgage, car, or any of a variety
of other expenses, it can seem like an easy decision to stop
paying the premiums on your life-insurance policy or making
contributions to your retirement savings plan. By purchasing
a policy with waiver-of-premium protection, you can ensure that
these investments are continued, and that your family is protected.

Retirement Rider

Because personal disability benefits from a privately purchased
plan are tax-free, the money you receive is considered unearned
income. However, only earned income can be put towards a retirement savings plan. As a result, if your disability plan provides
your only source of income, you will not be able to contribute
any money to a retirement savings plan. It is now possible to
purchase a retirement rider, which will contribute to your retirement fund for every month that you are unable to work because
of disability. This can be a very effective complement to your disability plan, and can ensure that your retirement fund will be
maintained and protected.

Children's Rider

If your child experiences a disability, the costs can also be astronomical. To protect yourself against this financial burden, you
can insure your children for an additional premium. If you have

adopted children, it is important that your policy specifies that they will also be covered. If this provision is included in your policy, it will ensure that your children obtain the type of care they need.

Sickness Wording
Some policies will not cover pre-existing conditions that are not diagnosed until after you purchased your policy. If a medical examination reveals that your illness (e.g., a slowly developing tumour) developed prior to the date that the policy came into force, it will not pay, even if you received a clean bill of health when you purchased the policy. If you purchase insurance with "sickness wording" that defines sickness as "a disease or disorder that first becomes apparent while this policy is in effect," you can protect yourself, and ensure that your benefits are paid in full.

Supplementary Disability Insurance
Even if your employer or association automatically provides disability insurance, you should always examine the quality of the plan. If the definition of disability is not comprehensive, or if the benefit plan is insufficient or not to your satisfaction, you can purchase a contract that will complement your work plan and assume the payment of benefits when the group or association plan ceases. It may be wise to get advice from a professional when purchasing a second policy. Some policies require the deduction of other disability payments. As a result, you may be left with less insurance than you think, and it will be the insurance company, not you, that benefits from your decision.

Brian
Brian worked for more than fourteen years as a production manager at a vegetable-packing plant. His duties ranged from

supervision to maintenance. In October 1995, at the age of fifty-six, Brian had a stroke. From then until April 1996, his company policy provided short-term disability benefits. From April 1996 to April 1998, the long-term disability (LTD) benefits, which paid Brian 60 percent of his net income, took over. This two-year term is standard in most group LTD plans. This amount was taxable, since the premiums were paid by the employer as part of the group LTD plan. As a result, Brian's real income dropped to approximately 50 percent of his pre-disability income. Fortunately, his employer continued his health and dental coverage while he received disability benefits.

A few months before the end of the two-year LTD period, Brian received a letter from his insurance company informing him that his case was under review. If the review indicated that it would be medically possible for him to do any job for which he was reasonably qualified, given his education, training, and experience, his benefits would terminate, whether there was a job available or not.

What options did Brian have?

1. **Could he return to his original job?** No. Balance problems prevented him from returning.
2. **Could the company provide him with another opportunity?** No. There were no openings available, so the company was not required to provide another job.
3. **Could he take early retirement?** Yes. But early retirement would have caused Brian major financial losses, as his retirement plan heavily penalized early withdrawal. His immediate financial obligations made this impossible.
4. **Could he find a new job?** Brian was unlikely to find a new company that would be willing to train and hire someone at his age.

Clearly, Brian faced serious financial problems as soon as he was diagnosed as being able to work. What could he have done differently? He should have considered group top-up or group offset insurance. These plans would have provided an increase in benefits (tax-free) or a continuation in the benefits of his group plan. Another option would have been a private personal plan that would kick in after a two-year waiting period. These plans can be purchased on a five- to ten-year basis, or until age sixty-five.

LIFE INSURANCE

If you don't have life insurance when you experience a disability, your chances of being able to purchase a plan are very slim. Ideally, you would have an adequate amount of life insurance before the disability occurs, but this rarely happens. The best way to ensure that you have access to adequate life insurance is to purchase a small policy (even if you feel that it may not be necessary at this point in your life) and include a future insurability option. This will allow you to purchase additional life insurance even when your health status would normally prevent you from doing so. The waiver-of-premium option is also worth considering.

Some life-insurance policies can also be used during times of disability. A life-insurance policy with cash values built up inside the plan can be accessed if needed. You can get a significant percentage of your life insurance paid out before your death to help cover expenses.

A recent innovation in the field of life insurance permits people who have been diagnosed with a terminal illness to sell their policies back to the insurance company or to speculative investors. The company or the investors then pay out a portion of the benefit in advance and keep the remainder of the policy as the cost of doing business. This procedure has proven very helpful for people with disabilities who need quick access to a large amount of money to take care of debts, cover the cost of care, or fulfil their wishes before they die. This option is only for people who are diagnosed with conditions that will be fatal in the short term (usually three to six months). If there is a chance that your condition will go into remission or that you may live for an extended period of time, this option should not be considered.

CRITICAL CARE/CRITICAL ILLNESS INSURANCE

We all know someone who has contracted a life-altering illness and survived. Although the chance of being diagnosed with a critical illness is increasing, medical advances are enabling more people to survive major health catastrophes. In fact, premature death levels have been falling dramatically in recent years, while critical-illness diagnoses have increased by approximately 55 percent in the past twenty-five years. Too many survivors are unprepared for the costs and pressures of such a crisis. Critical-illness insurance is designed to help you financially, by providing a lump-sum payment of between $10,000 and $1 million, tax-free, if you survive for thirty days after being diagnosed with an illness designated in the contract. If you do not survive for thirty days, however, your estate will not receive any benefits.

A contract can be designed to cover such conditions as heart attack, stroke, life-threatening cancer, coronary-artery bypass surgery, paralysis, blindness, deafness, kidney failure, multiple sclerosis, major organ transplant, Alzheimer's disease, Parkinson's disease, coma, loss of speech, and severe burns. It is even possible to tailor a plan to match your family's medical history, although this may be more expensive than a standard plan.

Any one of these illnesses could threaten both your lifestyle and your security, necessitating private nursing care; a reduction or permanent loss of income; a change in profession; and additional costs for child care, medical equipment, home retrofitting, relocation, and so forth. Coping with the physical aspects of a severe illness or accident is hard enough without a host of other pressures to distract you. You want to be able to focus your energy on healing and rehabilitating, not on finding a way to meet your mortgage or debt payments.

Although critical-illness insurance is not appropriate for everyone, it does provide several distinct benefits that other forms of insurance do not. Proponents of critical-illness insurance frame the issue in this fashion: If you owned an insurance policy that paid you a benefit if you contracted a disability, at what point during the disability would you want to be paid? (a) When the disability killed you; (b) when the disability prevented you from working; or (c) when the disability was diagnosed. Unlike life insurance, which covers you only in the event of your death, or disability insurance, which pays out benefits only for a limited period of time, critical-illness insurance can be used immediately for any purpose, and it is paid in full if you survive thirty days past diagnosis.

This type of coverage has risen to prominence in North America only in the 1990s, but its popularity is growing. Eligibility for coverage is based on your health alone. Unlike disability insurance, for which you need an earned income, critical-illness insurance can fill the void for the homemaker or business owner who does not earn an income, or who cannot show an earned income because their expenses offset their revenues.

There are several useful features built into critical-care insurance:

- If you die before becoming critically ill, most insurance companies will return all or a significant portion of your premiums as a form of life insurance. In this scenario, the consumer will always benefit. If you contract a critical illness, the benefit will be paid. If you die before the waiting period is over, or if you die without experiencing a critical illness, then your beneficiary will receive the payout.

- Children can also be included on a parent's critical-illness contract. If a child contracts an illness, money will be made available to provide them with the special care the child needed.

- The person insured can also name a charity to be the recipient of a contribution of approximately $500 from the insurance company, to aid in finding a cure for his disease.

BUSINESS INSURANCE

A disability that prevents you from working, even if it is for only a few months, can be especially devastating if you're a professional or a small-business owner who does not have adequate protection. Most business owners carry a significant debt and are responsible for staff, equipment, and leases; in some cases, they have clients or patients to whom they must deliver a service. A disability that disrupts service can lead to a significant loss of revenue, and even bankruptcy, if the individual is not protected. A private business (or medical/legal/dental practice) can be fully protected with a disability-income program that contains a number of provisions.

Business Overhead Insurance

If you encounter a disability that prevents you from performing the necessary functions of your daily business, business overhead insurance will allow you to pay your lease, debts, and other short-term expenses without fear of bankruptcy or default. Business overhead insurance will enable you to keep your staff, have sufficient time to evaluate and sell your assets or practice, and ensure that you do not have to cope with the responsibility of managing everything on your own when you are ill, which can compound the problem.

A policy that covers your overhead costs will benefit you and your employees. Insurance coverage will enable you to keep staff on the payroll until you are able to return to work, at which point you can start up again at full efficiency. If your disability prevents you from working only over the short term, it is usually cheaper to maintain your staff and then return to work six, eight, or ten months later than it is to let them go and then have to find and train new staff. Overhead insurance can also provide your employees with time to find alternate employment, or allow you to showcase your staff to a prospective buyer as an added asset of your company.

Another reason to buy business overhead protection is that it is tax-deductible. Even if you are just starting out, it is worthwhile to invest in a policy that can protect your business from potential disaster. Although it may stretch your budget over the short term, it is a wise investment over the long term. There are several other components to a comprehensive plan to protect your business from the impact of disability. The first is called key person insurance.

Key Person Insurance
Key person insurance reimburses your company for lost revenues and retraining costs if a key employee becomes sick or injured. The loss of a partner can prevent expansion, decrease productivity, increase expenses, erode consumer confidence, lower staff morale, and lead to increased pressure from banks and creditors. You can also buy key person insurance to protect you in the event that a partner dies. The insurance will ensure that you

have sufficient funds to keep your business going. Buy-sell protection is another way to guard your business in the event that you or your partner suffers a serious disability.

Buy-Sell Protection

If you are forced to sell your company after your partner suffers a disability, you may have to accept less than the market value or sell out to a new partner you don't want to work with. You may also be unable to support your share of the business, which can potentially cause bankruptcy. A pre-arranged buy-sell agreement with a partner or a third party can avoid all of these problems. It can save you significant time and worry, and can ensure that you will obtain fair value for your business.

HOW MUCH INSURANCE DO I NEED?

Disability-insurance premiums can cost 2 to 4 percent of your annual earned income. The premiums are not cheap, but when it comes to the quality of the contract, you get what you pay for! The cost of the premiums also pales in comparison to the costs of not being covered. All in all, it is certainly a reasonable investment.

A capital needs analysis is the most accurate way to determine how much life insurance you need. This analysis compares your assets with your debts, and considers the income your family or business will require in the event of death or disability. This "capital amount" also takes into account relevant rates of interest and inflation. These three case studies illustrate how much coverage people at certain levels of income might purchase.

If You Make $30,000

A person earning $30,000, married, with one child, should primarily be concerned with insuring all of his debts and having sufficient capital to pay for funeral expenses. If this person has a family who is dependent on his income for day-to-day living, then a capital needs analysis should be conducted to determine how much capital is required to ensure that the family's living arrangements do not have to be altered. For this level of income, coverage of between $50,000 to $200,000 is appropriate.

If this person has benefits available through his employer, the disability benefit should be adequate to insure against sickness or injury. Although the definition of disability will probably not be liberal, it is unlikely that an individual earning this amount of income will have the means to complement their group insurance with an individual disability policy.

If this person is self-employed or on contract, then a disability contract should be purchased that will insure his minimal level of monthly expenses. If it is affordable, he should ensure the maximum amount. If someone is not eligible for disability insurance, or if she is able to afford an extra premium, she should consider purchasing critical-illness insurance.

If You Make $50,000

A person earning approximately $50,000 a year should have all debts insured and consider providing additional income to his family in the event of his death, as the individual's salary is likely to be an essential part of the family's disposable income. A benefits level of $200,000 to $500,000 is appropriate. A rule of thumb for life insurance is to have $200,000 of coverage on the life of the primary income earner for each child in the family.

With this level of income, disability insurance is a must. Even if coverage is offered through an employer, complementing the base coverage with an individual policy should be considered if it is affordable. Critical-illness coverage should also be considered as part of an insurance portfolio. Purchasing enough to pay off a mortgage or to provide for home renovations or nursing assistance is also a worthy idea ($100,000 to $200,000 of coverage is appropriate).

If You Make $100,000

This person should have all debts insured against death and have enough life insurance to keep his family in their current living arrangement ($500,000 to $1 million of coverage is appropriate, but a capital needs analysis will determine a more specific amount).

Any group policy should be investigated to determine its maximum amount. Most group plans will pay a maximum of $2,500 to $3,000 per month for a disability claim, even if 67 percent of the employee's income is greater than this amount. The employee should top up his disability policy with individual coverage that will not only provide him with the appropriate benefits, but also give him a better definition of disability. Critical-illness coverage should be incorporated into the insurance portfolio. Purchasing sufficient coverage to pay off a mortgage and provide for home renovations and nursing assistance should also be considered ($200,000 to $500,000 of coverage).

BUILDING A FINANCIAL PLANNING TEAM

Few people are experts in financial planning, disability planning, legal planning, and risk assessment. Even if you have experience in some of these areas, it is a good idea to consult with professionals to ensure that you have developed a comprehensive plan. Some of the professionals who can contribute to the development of your plan include insurance agents, accountants, bank managers, attorneys, and financial planners.

Once you have decided on the list of professional services you require, these strategies can help you put together an effective planning team.

- **Recommendations.** Seek advice from friends, colleagues, and acquaintances on their experience with various professionals. You should also check with the local Better Business Bureau. They will be able to confirm the reputations of many of the companies and individuals whose services you are considering.
- **Deal with an established company.** Avoid groups offering deals or guarantees that seem too good to be true. Companies that have established records of providing sound financial advice will almost always represent your interests with integrity.
- **Shop around.** When you are considering a lifelong investment in something as important as a disability-protection plan, do not commit yourself to a particular supplier in advance. It is always a prudent idea to consult with a number of reputable representatives. This will ensure that you are exposed to a wide range of options. In addition, the pressures of competition may enable you to purchase your protection at a more reasonable rate.
- **Select your broker carefully.** Independent agents canvass the market for the best possible plans for their clients, for a set fee. Independent agents are very efficient, and they save you from having to compare all the policies on your own. Some experts consider independent agents to be more objective, because they are willing to examine the entire range of policies on the market, rather than only those offered by a specific firm.
- **Look for discounts.** Agents who work for a specific company are often able to obtain coverage at a lower rate than an independent agent. Company brokers are also supported by the credibility of their institutions. We have consulted with both independent and company represen-

tatives while researching this book, and both options can provide satisfactory results. The quality of the individual should be the determining factor.

Dealing with an Agent

When you purchase insurance, there are a number of steps you can take to make sure that you get what need.

Be Prepared

If you know exactly what you want to protect before you go to an agent, the process can go much more quickly and smoothly. If you are organized, you can inform your agent of the features you need and how much you are able to spend. If you present an agent with your clearly established priorities, it is unlikely that you will be bombarded with a range of options that don't interest you, or that you may not need.

Be Open to Advice

Although you should be well prepared and have a good idea of what you are going to buy when you enter an insurance office, try to remain open to the agent's advice. You are dealing with professionals, the vast majority of whom are honest and scrupulous. Even if you have done a good job preparing yourself, an agent will still have a more comprehensive knowledge of the range of policy options, and he may be able to provide you with some very valuable advice. This could entail identifying an aspect of coverage that you might have missed, or explaining how a variety of options can be configured to meet your needs. Endeavour to work in co-operation with financial-planning professionals, while keeping in mind that you have the final say.

Know Exactly What You Are Buying

This may be the single most important thing to remember when purchasing insurance. Read and understand your entire policy! Too many people encounter a nasty surprise when they submit a claim and discover that their coverage does not entitle them to certain benefits. *Always read the fine print to make sure that there are no undesirable exemptions in your policies.*

Reading the fine print is particularly important when buying insurance on a debt or mortgage. If you aren't careful, you may find some real zingers in those policies. The "previous health problems" section is very often not read and not filled in properly. This can mean that there will be no payment on the policy. People are especially neglectful about reading these sections because they are more concerned about the cost and have probably already signed numerous documents.

The fine print will tell you:

1. exactly which disabilities you are protected from and those from which you are not;
2. the amount and duration of the benefits you will receive;
3. what, if any, exemptions apply (i.e., disabilities caused by drunk driving, self-inflicted wounds, piloting a plane, or performing any other "dangerous" activity);
4. if the policy covers all disabilities that first become apparent while the policy is in force, or only those that developed after the policy was purchased;
5. the details of the company's cancellation policies;
6. exactly when the policy comes into play.

Go over each of these areas in great detail with your agent. Don't feel shy about asking for a detailed examination of your contract, and don't feel that you are imposing on him — it is his job. If an agent is unwilling to explain everything in your contract to you, you should refuse to purchase the policy and tell him that you will take your business elsewhere.

Regularly Review and Update Your Coverage
If you get married or have children, or get a raise at work, your needs and priorities will change. You may have new investments you want to protect (a college fund, a retirement savings plan, etc.), and you will want to make sure that your level of coverage does not lag behind your income. Review your insurance portfolio with your agent at least once a year, as well as every time your status changes. Review your investments at least every six months.

Learn About Your Prospective Company
By asking your agent a few simple questions, you can gauge the integrity of the company whose policy you are considering. Ask your agent:

1. How many policies does the company sell on an annual basis?
2. How many policies does your company pay out each year?
3. How many claims are paid out, in comparison to the number of claims that are made?
4. May I see some examples of how your company has followed up on recent claims?

If your questions are answered in a forthright manner, you can be reasonably sure that you are dealing with a reliable firm. In particular, it is desirable to find a firm that pays out benefits on a high percentage of claims.

CONCLUSION

This chapter has explained the basic components of an effective financial-protection plan, and has described how to go about building a plan, what features you should look for, and which pitfalls you should avoid. By consulting with a financial planner and carefully examining all your options, you can ensure that your future and that of your family are financially secure. Most disability plans do not have all of the features we have described. Tailor a plan to meet your needs.

When most people are establishing their careers and having families they underestimate the value of protecting themselves against disability. They are unaware of the resources that are available to provide stability and security in the event of a crisis. A proper insurance plan is one of these vital resources. Legal planning is another important one. It can help to ensure continuity and stability at a time when you may be vulnerable. In the next chapter we will discuss legal protection for disability, and how to file an insurance claim.

Ensuring Your Legal Protection and Filing a Claim

INTRODUCTION

In addition to your long-term concerns about health, discrimination, and returning to work, you may have legal problems following the onset of disability. If you have not planned for these, they can exact high legal, financial, and emotional costs. These problems can include confusion over your medical care, disputes over the management of financial resources and assets, and questions about whether you should continue with life support or participate in organ donation.

These problems can easily be avoided by designating powers of attorney for property and for personal care. Sometimes one person can fulfil both roles.

POWER OF ATTORNEY FOR PROPERTY

To ensure honest and professional management of your property and income if you are incapacitated, it is wise to give a trusted individual power of attorney over your property. Power of attorney grants the "attorney" (who does not have to be a lawyer) the power to do everything that you, the "donor," might have done. Any decisions about the property are deemed to be made with the donor's consent. If the power is defined as general, then the attorney has complete freedom to do everything that you would have done in financial matters, except make a will. If the power is specific, he may be limited to dealing with particular real-estate holdings or bank accounts. The attorney can be any mentally competent person who has reached the age of majority and is prepared to take on the responsibility of managing your affairs (without taking personal advantage).

The person or firm that you choose to hold this power should be trustworthy and competent. You can give power of attorney over property to a relative, but this may expose them to family conflicts. If a neutral third party is involved, it is unlikely that there will be accusations of favouritism, and bitter family disputes can sometimes be avoided. If a family member feels comfortable with assuming the responsibility, however, she can often be just as effective as a professional. This will save you the cost of hiring an attorney, but you should be aware of the risks. Your attorney should be familiar with financial matters, so she will be able to properly manage your affairs.

A power of attorney is valid only when signed and dated by the donor and witnessed by a specific number of people (which varies from place to place). There may be restrictions on who can be a witness — a spouse or relative of the donor may not be eligible. In some states and provinces, witnesses under the age of majority are ineligible. You can designate someone as your attorney without their knowledge, but it is always a good idea to gain their consent before you act. Because the law varies from state to state, province to province, it is advisable to obtain legal advice before executing any power of attorney.

Canada and the U.S. now allow enduring powers of attorney for property. "Enduring" means that the power of attorney will survive the donor's subsequent mental incompetence, but only if the donor explicitly makes this provision in the document itself. If you rely on a power of attorney document, check the wording to make sure that the "mental incapacity" provision is included. Some jurisdictions have only recently allowed this measure, and older documents may be out of date.

You can revoke the power of attorney at any time, as long as you are mentally capable. The law may vary from place to place, but if you make the decision to revoke your power of attorney, do so in writing, retrieve the original power of attorney document, and destroy it. It is a good idea not to make any copies of the original document. If several copies of the power of attorney exist, it may be difficult to change it, or you may have two powers of attorney in conflict. If there is only one copy, you can simply destroy the document to revoke it.

Review your powers of attorney regularly, especially after you marry, separate, or divorce, or if you experience a significant change in health or financial circumstances. Inform your close relatives and business associates that you have created a power of attorney, so they know who to consult in the event of a serious disability. You do not need to inform them of the contents of the document. If you decide to make copies of the power of attorney, keep a list of the people to whom you have given one alongside your own copy of the document.

A power of attorney for property is limited to making decisions about the financial management of your affairs. A person with power of attorney for property cannot make decisions about your personal care unless you sign a separate personal care document.

POWER OF ATTORNEY FOR PERSONAL CARE

The power of attorney for personal care is very similar to the power of attorney for property. Sometimes known as a living will, it allows you to designate a proxy who can make decisions for you when you are no longer mentally or physically capable. These decisions may include where you will live, what medical treatment you will receive, how far caregivers should go to resuscitate you or prolong your life, the composition of your diet, and other issues.

A power of attorney for personal care will ensure that conflict or disagreement among your family members over your wishes is minimized, as it explicitly spells out what measures you do or do not want performed. A living will is an excellent way to participate in your own care, and to ensure that your wishes are respected. If a patient becomes seriously ill and doctors are forced to make a decision about life support without a legal document, the patient's wishes will not necessarily be respected. If there is no living will, a patient who has expressed her desire not to have her life artificially prolonged may not have her wishes respected, especially if another family member wants to keep her alive. Conflicts over these issues have led to expensive and divisive legal battles.

The attorney for personal care does not have to be the same person as the attorney for property. In fact, in some cases they should not be, as these people perform very different roles. Choose the agent of your power of attorney for personal care very carefully. Because the person making these decisions may be responsible for your life or death, they should know you very well, and you should share similar values. Only designate someone who is willing to take on this responsibility, and who has the time and interest to fulfil her duties properly as your attorney.

Discuss your wishes in detail with the attorney for personal care and close family members. You may have different directives depending on the condition, so it is essential that you spell out your wishes in great detail, in order to avoid any confusion. For example, if you are in a coma that may be only temporary, you probably want doctors to do everything possible to keep you alive. On the other hand, if you are in a coma from which there is little or no chance of recovery, you may want life support to be discontinued. The decision to continue life support may also have implications for your finances or insurance policies. Be aware of all of these factors before you commit to a decision. Having the wrong outcome because you did not make your preferences clear can be tragic.

Some jurisdictions will not recognize all of the provisions of living wills. Specifically, they may refuse to consider the directive not to resuscitate when dying, or the one to turn off respirators. Other provisions based on religious beliefs, such as the refusal to accept blood transfusions, may be overruled by the courts. If you reside in one of these jurisdictions, the best way to ensure that your wishes are respected is to make them very well known to your friends, family, and caregivers, and to express them clearly in your powers of attorney.

The power of attorney for personal care is designated in the same fashion as the power of attorney for property, and it can be revoked as long as you are mentally competent. There may be some restrictions placed on who you can select, so as to avoid a conflict of interest. Those excluded may include nursing home staff, doctors, nurses, landlords, or others. Spouses or partners are not excluded.

THE IMPORTANCE OF A LEGAL WILL

It is also important to have a legal will to ensure that your wishes are followed in the event of your death. If you do not have a will, the government will usually distribute your assets in a specific pattern according to applicable legislation. The absence of a will can also lead to conflict between family members and friends. Assets may be used for legal fees instead of being distributed as benefits. A lawyer can help you draw up a will within a very short period of time, and she can help to minimize the tax on the estate. It is worth this small investment to provide your family with security.

Your executor, the person who oversees your estate, should be someone you trust, either a family member or a professional, such as a lawyer or the person exercising your power of attorney. Sometimes it is a good idea to appoint co-executors, one family member and one professional. If your will is relatively complex, it may be wise to hire a professional executor who fully understands all of the provisions. A financial planner and a lawyer who specializes in estate law can help you determine how best to structure your will. The proper legal preparation can alleviate much of the trauma that accompanies death and disability.

FILING A CLAIM

Many people think that as long as they have disability coverage, they will be automatically covered in the event of an accident or illness. This is not always the case! Insurance companies examine every claim for benefits very carefully. Sometimes claims are paid promptly, but in other cases, especially those that involve large payouts, the payment of benefits can be delayed for months. Some legitimate claims are challenged and even denied. If you follow recommended procedures, you can ensure that your claim will be processed as quickly as possible. Here are some suggestions on how to make an effective claim.

Obtain a Diagnosis

If you are unable to work because of a disability, it is imperative that you get an accurate medical diagnosis as soon as possible. Apart from the proven medical benefits of swift diagnosis, you will not be eligible to receive any benefits until you have established the medical legitimacy of your claim. If the doctor's diagnosis indicates that you should file a claim, proceed directly to a lawyer who specializes in representing clients in cases dealing with insurance companies.

The Importance of Consulting a Specialist

It is always a good idea to get your lawyer (preferably a specialist in personal-injury law) to file your claim and handle all of the necessary interactions with the insurance company. There are a number of benefits to using an established personal-injury lawyer.

1. Your lawyer will be familiar with all of the procedures that must be completed in order to file a claim. As a result, he will probably be able to help you avoid any technical delays in receiving your payment.
2. He will be a strong advocate on your behalf.
3. He will be able to recognize the difference between a good offer and a bad offer.
4. He will not be intimidated.
5. He will be able to arrange an independent assessment of your disability. Most personal-injury lawyers work with professional assessors (specialists in evaluating the short- and long-term costs associated with disability) who can help you determine what your needs will be so you can make an accurate claim. Most people have little idea of what the total cost of their disability will be. By going

to specialists, you ensure that all of your possible costs will be identified.

6. After the costs have been determined, your lawyer will ensure that all relevant documents are included when he files a claim on your behalf.

Physical Re-examination

Once you have filed your claim, the insurance company may wish to have you re-examined by their own physicians and assessors. Consent to these examinations, as well as to any other reasonable requests the insurance company makes, assuming that is the advice of your lawyer. As long as your policy was underwritten and you are being honest, you should have little to worry about.

Sometimes your doctors and the insurance doctors will make competing statements. In most cases, this means that the insurance company's doctors are minimizing the extent of your injuries and the cost of your care. These conflicts can result in extensive delays, and sometimes even court battles. As long as you are being honest and are effectively represented, you should not back down in the face of competing medical claims. Usually a compromise can be reached, and even if a court case is necessary, the courts will generally support a legitimate claim.

Evaluating an Offer

After its doctors have performed an assessment, the insurance company will make an offer, either to you or to your lawyer. Most reputable companies will always go through your lawyer. Indeed, employees may be reprimanded if they deal directly with a claimant when the claimant has a lawyer. They should accept that you have designated the lawyer as your spokesperson, and respect that relationship.

Some companies have been known to make offers directly to the claimant without the lawyer's knowledge. These offers may seem like a lot of money, but they are usually far lower than could otherwise be claimed. Often they are made to worried clients who are experiencing financial difficulties in addition to the stress of a disability. Frequently, people will jump at the first offer, which seems generous and provides the immediate opportunity to pay debts and bills. It is always unethical, and in many jurisdictions illegal, for an insurance company to bypass a legal representative when settling a claim. Nonetheless, it does occur. If you find yourself in this situation, immediately refer the insurance representative to your attorney. Refuse to sign any agreement that is not approved by your legal representative.

There have been numerous instances of people being approached by insurance companies and signing away claims for all future benefits in exchange for a one-time payout that seemed generous. I recently spoke to a personal-injury lawyer who told me of a client who accepted a single, final payout of $20,000 when her needs indicated that she might have been entitled to tens of thousands more. Said this lawyer, "She has no idea of what her long-term expenses will be. I am sure that I could have easily obtained over $200,000 for my client."

The moral is to be tough. Don't feel hurt or offended if an insurance company aggressively examines your claim. This is simply a part of their business. Understandably, they do not want to be ripped off. In some instances, however, people encounter problems when making their claims. Insurance companies have tremendous resources, and sometimes claimants feel like David facing Goliath. However, if you have been honest with your insurers, have designed an appropriate plan, and are well represented, your claim should be paid.

Sheila

Sheila was a thirty-five-year-old woman from Montreal who worked as a veterinarian. She had owned a private disability policy for ten years, because her workplace did not have long-term group insurance. She became pregnant, and over the course of her pregnancy considered cancelling her policy to help pay for the costs of her baby. Ultimately, she decided not to. Despite some complications, she delivered a healthy baby. While on maternity leave, however, she developed a severe case of rheumatoid arthritis. She was unable to work for one year because of her disability.

As soon as she learned of her medical problems, she contacted her insurance agent. He started to fill out the complicated but necessary paperwork, and referred her to two physicians. Her general practitioner and her specialist were each required to write two reports. The insurance company made requests for more extensive information about her condition, and she was required to undergo quarterly medical assessments. This woman faced a thirty-day waiting period before she received any benefits from her policy, and a total of three months passed before her first cheque arrived.

Her plan called for coverage of $2,000 per month. With this, she was able to maintain her standard of living until she was healthy enough to return to work. Because she had a personal policy on which she paid the premiums, her benefits were 100 percent tax-free. Any policy on which you (rather than an employer) pay the premiums will provide benefits without any tax.

PROBLEMS WITH FILING A CLAIM

Resistance to Diagnosis

Many people who have legitimate disabilities find it difficult to have their insurance company or employer accept the diagnosis of the medical condition that is keeping them from work. Back pain, repetitive strain injury, chronic fatigue syndrome, post-traumatic stress syndrome, and many other conditions are not always recognized as legitimate, and their victims are often denied the appropriate compensation or treatment.

There are three main reasons why firms resist paying claims. The first is financial. To save funds, an employer and its insurer may challenge the legitimacy of a diagnosis or interpret a claim in such a way as to exclude the condition from coverage. For example, if a policy covers disability resulting from physical stress but not psychological stress, an organization may decide to categorize post-traumatic stress syndrome (PTSS) as a psychological condition, thus exempting the employer and the insurance company from financial responsibility. Numerous police officers have been denied benefits on these grounds. Other individuals whose employment has exposed them to dangerous situations have experienced similar treatment. Fortunately, in recent years, PTSS has been recognized as a legitimate physical and psychological condition, and more companies are providing compensation.

Resistance to payment can also stem from a genuine disagreement over the validity of a condition. This challenge can take clinical and individual forms. Clinical challenges occur when an institution refuses, or is reluctant to acknowledge, the legitimacy of the claims of an individual experiencing a specific disability. Usually these are invisible disabilities. For example, many people who experience whiplash are unable to work because of pain, loss of balance, loss of the ability to concentrate, and a host of other continuing symptoms. Because it is an "invisible" disability, however, many employers and insurance companies are reluctant to acknowledge its validity as a clinical condition that requires compensation. Such conditions may not be included in long-term disability coverage. To provide yourself with comprehensive disability coverage, you may have to purchase additional insurance.

Resistance to payment can also occur when an institution questions the validity of an individual's claim. Essentially, they will suggest that you are faking it. Insurance fraud does occur, and this has led to suspicion on the part of payers. Their increased vigilance has unfortunately caused extended delays for many people with real disabilities, and some have even been deprived of their benefits. If you face this sort of discrimination, it may be necessary to pursue legal action.

Sometimes two doctors will make different diagnoses of the same patient. Physicians representing insurance companies are sometimes inclined to attribute a patient's suffering to a condition that traditionally would not require compensation, while the patient's physician or a third party may issue a diagnosis that would lead to greater compensation. This can be seen in the story of a friend of mine who has had a hearing impairment since birth. Richard graduated from university with a degree in pharmacy, and worked for fifteen years as a pharmacist. In the last three years he worked, his hearing worsened, to the point that he was no longer able to understand instructions given over the telephone, and he was unable to hear many orders and requests placed by customers. This made it extremely difficult for him to continue his practice, and even caused him to make several unintentional mistakes while performing his duties. After a full evaluation from his audiologist, he made a claim for disability benefits, which was denied following a lengthy examination by the insurance company. After a long and expensive court battle, the pharmacist was able to demonstrate the legitimacy of his claim, and he has been on full disability ever since. If you are pressing for the recognition of a genuine disability, the legal system can help get your needs addressed.

Sometimes, given the same diagnosis, two doctors may still differ on its impact on an individual. Insurance companies will sometimes argue that because patients with conditions similar to yours are functioning well, you should not be entitled to benefits. For example, there have been many court cases involving rheumatism and arthritis and their role in limiting an individual's capacity to function in her job. The cases are decided on the degree of incapacitation, the extent of the plan's coverage, and the length of an individual's working career. It is always better to try to reach a settlement, but if you are making a legitimate claim and have strong evidence to support your position, the courts will usually decide in your favour.

Resistance to Payment of Benefits

Most people assume that they will be covered by their long-term disability insurance, but many find that it is very difficult, if not impossible, to obtain the benefits to which they feel they are entitled. Cases often hinge on the legal and medical definitions of "disability" and "incapacitation." For example, two parties may acknowledge that an individual has carpal tunnel syndrome. However, the parties may disagree over the extent of the incapacity. The employer may argue that the individual is not incapacitated, because others experiencing a similar condition continue to work. The employer may be willing to purchase special adaptive equipment and allow for creative work schedules and physiotherapy, but he may refuse to pay for disability leave.

In addition to disagreements over the level of incapacity, parties may disagree over whether a medical condition constitutes a disability at all. A dentist experienced the severe deterioration of both knees at the age of fifty-two. The pain increased to the point where he was unable to walk or stand without excruciating pain. Although he still had the manual dexterity and skill to carry out his technical duties, he had to be on his feet all day and the pain made it very difficult for him to continue working. He had knee replacements in an attempt to eliminate the pain, but the surgery was only partially successful, and he was unable to continue his practice. Although he had always paid his long-term disability premiums, he had to go through a four-year legal battle to obtain his benefits. His case illustrates that you should not take anything for granted. You may have to engage legal services to gain the benefits to which you are legally entitled!

MAKING THE MOST OF YOUR SETTLEMENT

When you make a successful insurance claim, or win a lawsuit that provides you with a significant cash award, keep in mind the intended purpose of the settlement and resist the temptation to spend the windfall unwisely. According to a study performed by the Rand Corporation, 69 percent of people who receive a financial windfall spend the money within three years, and in such a fashion that they are unable to take care of their future needs. This was the case whether the windfall came from the lottery, an inheritance, or a medical claim. When you receive a large sum of money, the temptation is to go on an extended vacation, purchase numerous luxury items, and disregard the principles of sound financial planning.

This type of behaviour can be very dangerous if you or a loved one have encountered a disability that has significant long-term costs. Because a one-time settlement is intended to last you the rest of your life, you may be out of luck if you waste it. Some people are very prudent and do not run into any difficulties, but for others, who may lack financial-planning skills, the consequences can be dire. Following the advice of a reputable financial planner is one way to protect yourself. Foregoing the traditional lump-sum payment for a "structured settlement" is another way to do it.

What Is a Structured Settlement?

A structured settlement is an alternative to the conventional lump-sum settlement: the traditional single payment is replaced with a series of periodic payments. This does not mean that structured settlements do not allow for lump-sum payments — in fact, a structured settlement can be shaped to meet the needs of each individual situation. Structured settlements can be formulated to allow "up-front" lump-sum payments, to allow income to be varied from year to year, to allow certain elements to be deferred from year to year, to allow for lump-sum benefits at various times in the future, and to allow for the escalation of payments in an effort to offset the effects of inflation.

Structured settlements are usually composed of two distinct elements: a cash portion paid up front and an annuity payment plan. The former is intended to pay for out-of-pocket expenses incurred prior to settlement, as well as any necessary capital expenditures such as modifications to vehicles or to the family home, legal fees, etc. The latter is designed to provide a series of payments (usually monthly) to meet your future financial needs. The fixed-income annuities provide a guaranteed income, and therefore your revenue will not be subject to the fluctuations of the stock market.

For example, if your disability necessitates the use of an electric wheelchair, which needs to be replaced every five years and costs up to $11,000 each time, a provision can be built into your settlement to provide the necessary additional revenue every five years. It is easier to plan for these capital investments in advance than to have to worry about how you will pay for each new expense.

Perhaps the most advantageous element of the structured settlement is how it is treated in the tax system. Most special and general damages received in personal-injury or accident cases are not subject to tax. Unfortunately, however, the income derived from these investments is taxed. Income generated by way of investment is tax-free only in a structured settlement, which is subject to a series of conditions that can be explained to you by your financial adviser. A structured settlement may not be right in all cases, but it is certainly an option that is worthy of consideration.

When a Structured Settlement Is Appropriate

A structured settlement may be appropriate if:

- your settlement is in excess of $50,000;
- you experienced serious bodily injury that will result in higher future care costs;
- you receive a future care claim or future lost income claim;
- multiple parties have a claim on the settlement;
- accident benefits are called for;
- an infant or young child is the recipient of the benefits (the return on investment in a structured settlement usually exceeds the interest earned on a lump sum held in trust);
- the beneficiary is financially unsophisticated and does not have the desire or knowledge to manage his own portfolio;
- the claimant wants a quick resolution to her claim (structured settlements are usually developed in a less adversarial fashion and lead to quicker resolutions than other settlements);
- the claimant is in a high tax bracket and would benefit from the tax-free income of a structured settlement.

CONCLUSION

Clearly expressing your wishes in a power of attorney or living will can save you and your family from a lot of uncertainty and confusion. If you experience a serious injury or illness, you and your family should be able to devote all of your time and energy to coping, not arguing over issues that could have been resolved by prior planning. You have to be tough when disability occurs. Don't allow anyone to push you around or dictate your future. Professional legal advice can ensure that you are the one in charge of the most important decisions about your medical care and finances. Legal advocates can also ensure that you receive your legitimate entitlement if you receive an insurance claim. Don't neglect this important source of personal protection.

PART

4

Resources

Chapter 14

Computers
and Disability

INTRODUCTION

The Internet has revolutionized the way information is disseminated in our society. The World Wide Web has emerged as a massive storehouse of information that allows anyone to perform research on virtually any topic in a matter of minutes. Information that used to be available only to experts is now available to the general public at the click of a button.

The Internet offers people with disabilities ready access to the latest information (and misinformation) concerning their conditions. For example, people living with chronic conditions such as diabetes or fibromyalgia can find out about the latest experimental techniques that are being developed to treat their conditions. This chapter includes case studies of three Internet searches by people who were recently diagnosed with a disability. These searches illustrate how to use the Internet to gain the information needed to make educated decisions about your plan of care. The case studies are not designed as step-by-step manuals for information gathering, but rather to illustrate the possibilities of the Internet as a research tool.

AVOIDING MISINFORMATION ON THE NET

It is important that anyone using the Internet as a source of information be aware that there is no limit to what can be published on it. Although there is a vast amount of valuable information available, there is also much misinformation to be avoided, because the Internet is very difficult to regulate. Don't be intimidated by media horror stories of fraud on the Net, but don't take anything published on the Internet as the gospel truth, either. Use the same critical thinking skills that you would apply to any medium to the Internet. Take the information that you learn on the Internet as a starting point and confirm it with outside research. Many people on the Net are just trying to make a quick buck, and they sometimes prey on the fears of innocent consumers.

The Internet is a hotbed of unconventional medical therapies that offer solutions for people suffering from "incurable" conditions. While these programs may occasionally provide genuine relief, it is important to be aware that some people on the Net make their living selling hope to patients at a time when they are most vulnerable. If you take a critical and objective view of the information you discover through your computer, and always confirm what you read with an independent source (i.e., your physician), there is almost nothing on the Internet that can hurt you. Nonetheless, always be wary of people who are "selling something." **Be very cautious if you plan to give out credit card numbers or any other information that could be misused.**

Information can be put on the Internet by private companies; governments; consumer advocacy groups; medical-research organizations; medical associations; private citizens; and medical and research journals. Some of the services provided on-line are available for a fee, and some are available only through educational institutions. You may be well served by beginning your search at a Web site created by or affiliated with a major and reputable organization in your area of interest. For example, someone from Toronto who had just suffered a mild stroke may decide to start looking for information at the Heart and Stroke Foundation of Canada Web site (www.hsf.ca). No matter where you begin, confirm the integrity of your source before you pursue any of the strategies you find.

SUPPORT OVER THE INTERNET

One of the most helpful features on the Internet is the availability of interactive on-line discussion groups, including list-servs, newsgroups, and chat rooms. These forums allow individuals to share information, coping strategies, and emotional support with people who have similar concerns. A list-serv is a distributed e-mail list on which members send a message to a central computer, and a copy is sent to all subscribers of the list. Newsgroups consist of messages posted to a central forum, where they can be read and responded to by anyone who visits the site, and chat rooms are live discussions (typed) in which anyone who logs on to a site can "talk" to someone in real time. You can post messages that outline your concerns or pose questions about your disability. Your message will be read by medical specialists and people from all over the world who share your disability, and who may be able to offer support or assistance. Typically, listservs are the most likely to be used or monitored by professionals, and chat rooms are the least likely.

The Internet is a unique resource for individuals who have conditions that occur so infrequently that support groups for them do not exist. If you have a very rare condition, posting messages to major disability sites can help you get in touch with people who share your situation. Some Web sites are dedicated to rare conditions, and may be of particular assistance.

GAINING ACCESS TO THE INTERNET

If you don't own your own computer, you can gain access to the Internet from libraries, Internet cafés, universities and colleges, elementary schools, high schools, computer stores, a friend's computer, and Internet service providers (ISPs). National ISPs include America Online, Compuserve, Prodigy, and Sympatico, and there are many ISPs at the local level as well. Full Internet access can cost as little as ten dollars per month. Paying for a couple of hours of access each month may be a worthwhile investment.

HOW TO USE THE INTERNET

We have included three case studies that illustrate how people living with disabilities have used the Internet to find information about their condition, and then have used that knowledge to gain some control over their treatment and care. First is a woman who was facing the possibility that she might have breast cancer. She used the Internet to help find answers to the questions that were foremost on her mind. It gave her access to a wide range of information in a short period of time, and that helped her to formulate the best questions to ask her doctor. Second is a case study of a man who was diagnosed with fibromyalgia. Although this is considered an incurable, chronic disease, he was able to use the Internet to find out about "alternative" treatments and to get support from others with the same condition. The third case study is a brief review of the ways in which an individual with quadraplegia gained information about coping with her condition.

Case Study: Breast Cancer and the Internet

This story describes how one woman used the Internet to seek answers to worrying questions about breast cancer.

I went to my family doctor because I noticed a dime-sized lump in my breast. He told me there was a good chance that the lump was malignant, as my grandmother had had breast cancer. My doctor made an appointment to have a biopsy done, then told me to go home and said we should wait until after we had the results before we talked about treatment options.

I decided to look on the World Wide Web to find out what I could about breast cancer. I particularly wanted answers to the following questions:

1. Will the biopsy procedure hurt?
2. What treatments are available for this type of breast cancer?
3. If I undergo surgery to remove the cancer, will I lose my whole breast?
4. Is there a danger that the cancer will spread to the rest of my body?
5. What are my chances of surviving breast cancer?

I went home, dialed up the Net, and launched my Web browser. I clicked on the Netsearch button on the Netscape Navigator toolbar to begin my search of the World Wide Web. Clicking this button sent me to the Netscape search page (http://home.netscape.com/escapes/search/netsearch), where I was able to choose from a number of search engines, including Lycos, Excite, Infoseek, and AltaVista. A search engine is a method of searching for key words that sorts the results according to your preferences. I didn't have any particular preference, so I used Lycos, which was the active engine at the time.

The Lycos search engine gave me the option of searching the whole World Wide Web using keywords, or narrowing my search into one of several pre-defined subject areas. There were over thirty choices, including Autos, Business, Careers, Health, Travel, and Women. I chose the Health subject area, but made a mental note to search under Women if Health did not have what I was looking for.

The Health search page was divided into a daily feature section, a community guides section, and a free services section. At the top of the page was another primary menu that offered more choices for narrowing my search. I did not find any leads about breast cancer under the specialized section, so I decided to look under the primary menu. The choices there included Fitness, Diseases, Women, Alternatives, Nutrition, and Men. I decided to continue my search for information concerning breast cancer by looking under the Diseases directory.

The Diseases directory contained three sections: a menu of more refined search parameters, a link to BarnesandNoble.com, and a special section on community guides. The community guides section listed links to information on a number of diseases, ranging from ALS to visual impairment. Unfortunately, breast cancer was not one of the choices. The Barnes and Noble site highlighted specific articles on a special topic. On the day I did my search, the topic was stress and the site provided links to articles dealing with stress management. Having not found any links dealing with breast cancer, I decided to look to the main menu and choose from the choices listed there. Topic choices included AIDS/HIV, Cancer, Drugs and Treatments, Mental Illness, and Substance Abuse. I clicked on the link marked Cancer and was taken to yet another part of the Lycos Web site.

The Cancer page had a list of cancer-related search parameters, which included Cancer Institutes, Cancer Patients, Hospices,

Chemotherapy, and Cancer Organizations. Breast Cancer was at the top of the list. After only three minutes of searching, I had found my first direct reference to breast cancer. After clicking on the Breast Cancer link, I was taken to a page that listed the top Web sites for breast cancer information. The number-one site had the headline "Mayo Doctors Downplay Mammogram False Alarms." Other hits included "2 Chicks, 2 Bikes, 1 Cause," Cancer Research Foundation of America, Breast Cancer Society of Canada, and Breast Cancer Doctor's Guide to the Internet.

I decided to make the Breast Cancer Society my first stop on the information superhighway. After approximately five minutes of searching the World Wide Web, I had found a page dedicated to information about breast cancer. The Breast Cancer Society's homepage is devoted to supporting victims of breast cancer and advocating for their rights. This page provided me with very little usable information about the nature of my disease, but it did help me by supplying a list of questions I could ask my doctor and by providing general information about the disease. This page was an excellent information source for people curious about breast cancer in general and for those diagnosed with the disease who already understand the medical issues involved. However, it was unable to answer all my questions, so I wanted to find another page with a more medical focus.

I decided to go back to my original list of hits at Lycos and look for a page that could help me answer my questions. One of the choices offered by my original search was the Breast Cancer Doctor's Guide to the Internet (http://www.pslgroup.com/ BREASTCANCER.HTM). I decided to visit this page because it looked like it was likely to have answers to my medical questions about breast cancer. After clicking around for a minute or two, however, I felt confused by the masses of information. The site was very big, and parts of it had nothing to do with breast cancer. I finally got to a list of articles about various drugs and their effectiveness, but they did very little to help me answer the questions I had set out to resolve by looking on the Internet.

I was having a hard time finding answers to specific questions, but I was exposed to a great deal of information about breast cancer that improved my general knowledge about the disease. I decided to direct my search towards my specific questions by using keywords. My first question was "Will the biopsy procedure hurt?" so I decide to type "breast biopsy" in the keyword search box at the top of the search page.

This produced a number of different hits, but the first few choices looked too medical and scientific. I finally chose a link marked "Breast Biopsy" from a page located at http://www.healthanswers.com. According to the information provided on this page, my doctor would use a local anesthetic, which would be somewhat painful when it was administered. The information stated that the procedure itself would be uncomfortable, but not painful, and that I would probably feel some tenderness afterwards.

By this point, I had been searching on the Internet for only twenty minutes, and I had already answered one of my questions. If I had used keyword searches right from the start, I would have answered all of my questions even faster. General searches are good for providing broad-based and reliable information, while keyword searches are a better way to find information on a specific topic.

Don't be afraid to "play around" on the Internet for a little while if you are not exactly sure what you are looking for. Spending thirty minutes or an hour moving from site to site without a specific plan can help you become more comfortable with the Internet and with the material that you will come across. Starting at a random site and searching in what seems like a haphazard pattern will often take you where you want to go.

Case Study: Fibromyalgia and the Internet

This is the story of how a man named Jerry used the Internet to help develop an alternate course of treatment for his disability.

In April 1997 I was diagnosed with fibromyalgia. I was told by my doctor, as well as by a few people I knew, that I would have this debilitating disease for the rest of my life — that fibromyalgia could not be cured. I chose not to accept such a dire prediction. There were many avenues I pursued in my quest for information, and one that was most helpful was searching on the Internet. This allowed me to connect with other people who suffered from the disease, as well as with a wide assortment of health-care practitioners and professionals.

Using the AltaVista search engine, I typed in "fibromyalgia" and punched the search button. There are many other excellent search engines, such as Lycos, Dejanews, Yahoo, and Web Crawler. Within moments, more than 4,000 hits on the disease were placed at my disposal. Some of the references were worthless, but many contained various first-person accounts of successful methods being used to combat the disease. In many instances, you could communicate directly with the individual whose story was posted on the Net.

My approach to evaluating their descriptions was based in part on whether they were selling something. If they were, I tended to dismiss their claims. If they were not, I continued "talking" to them via the Internet.

A large number of scholarly and not-so-scholarly articles were also placed at my disposal. I read many of these articles, though I tended to be somewhat more accepting of those that appeared in mainstream journals, and less accepting of those that appeared in one-time-only newsletters. Many of the latter were seeking to sell some miracle cure.

I would discuss with my doctor those articles that I found to be of merit. Fortunately, my doctor was open to naturopathic and homeopathic remedies. I cannot say that I am now permanently cured — perhaps the disease is only in remission, and I still have a way to go to rebuild my muscle strength — but the healing process is in full swing.

Case Study: Computers and Quadriplegia

This is the story of a woman named Vicki who has used computers extensively to help her cope with her disability.

I started using on-line services back in the days of 300 baud modems and monochrome screens. E-mail was not a household word and the Internet was still a government pet project. I was eleven or twelve then, and I found this means of communication fascinating. Here I was, in a distant suburb of Washington, D.C., talking to people in Wyoming, Alaska, and Germany — all at once.

My interest in computers kept growing. I taught myself what I could because PCs weren't quite mainstream and there weren't many classes available to young people. When I was in a car accident that left me with quadriplegia at the age of seventeen, however, computers quickly took over my life. They were no longer a hobby, but a necessary piece of equipment I needed to accomplish everyday tasks.

Now my computer is specifically adapted to my needs, with special software, voice activation, a headset mouse, and a smaller keyboard for typing with a mouth stick. I can use my computer and the Internet independently, as easily as those who operate a computer with their hands. I am now in college, studying English and creative writing. With my adapted system, I can navigate the Internet with ease, looking up information for research papers or downloading software to help me with my studies. E-mail plays a key role in helping me communicate with people when I am otherwise unable. If I am sick or run into complications (which so frequently haunt those of us with disabilities), I can e-mail my professors an explanation for my absence, or send them my completed assignments. Classmates use e-mail to keep me caught up with notes and assignments.

On-line communication is a great way to meet people. In the virtual world, you are faceless, ageless, sexless, and perhaps most important, without a disability. You are judged by your personality, not your looks or disability. E-mail keeps me in touch with family and friends. Here at college, I can talk to my family or my boyfriend whenever I want (and avoid the high phone bills).

I've even obtained a job via the Internet. I write reviews and news for the Baltimore section of MTV On-line. Since MTV is based in New York City, I communicate with my supervisor entirely through e-mail. Plus, my work is published on the Web. It's a great opportunity for an aspiring writer. Many company Web sites list their job openings. A good place to start is at the New Mobility Jobline at http://www.newmobility.com.

The Internet keeps me in touch with the world around me. Since my accident, I have had great difficulty reading the newspaper. The Internet has services (InfoBeat is a personal favourite) that e-mail the latest news, sports, entertainment, and weather right to your desktop. Reading by scrolling down a screen is much easier than trying to flip those large newspaper pages with a mouth stick. On-line communication and the Internet substantially lessen my day-to-day difficulties, and those seemingly insurmountable obstacles are more easily overcome.

CONCLUSION

Computers and the Internet provide vast opportunities for people both with and without disabilities to learn about health issues. The Internet has fed the public's growing demand for information about health and wellness issues, and it probably contains more raw material than any other source. This explosion in the amount of information available at the touch of a button has helped thousands of people with disabilities and their loved ones to become informed, proactive consumers of care. Appendix C provides you with a list of some of the most useful Web sites that can help you get started.

The Internet is an important resource for anyone who wants to become more knowledgeable about her condition. It can help to relieve uncertainty after an initial diagnosis, it can put you in touch with a warm and caring support network, and it can keep you up-to-date on recent medical advances. The Internet can complement any protection plan, and can help you take control of your care.

The Internet can also provide you with confidence. The Internet provides access to unlimited amounts of information, which you can use to build expertise on your condition. Developing an understanding of your condition and your options is one of the best ways to become more comfortable with your disability. Knowledge can minimize uncertainty and bring you the power to seek out new ideas and options, and to actively participate in your own care.

Appendix A

Sample Letters

INTRODUCTION

The following sample letters will help you build coalitions and gain access to the best opportunities and resources. You should send copies to all relevant individuals, and keep a copy on file for your personal records.

Sample Letter #1

This letter requests space in an independent living centre (ILC). It outlines a case where an entire family is looking into an ILC. Your letter should include the specific details of your condition, what your needs are, what contributions you can make to the ILC, and why you want to live in an ILC.

Dear Sir or Madam:

My name is _____ , and for the last five years I have been living with rheumatoid arthritis. During the last year and a half, it has become extremely difficult for me to live in my present rental accommodation. I am making a somewhat unusual request: I would like to acquire accommodation not only for myself, but also for my wife and seven-year-old child. I am no longer able to work, but my wife makes a satisfactory income.

I require accommodation that is close to public transportation, as I must make several trips every week to my physician and to two local rehabilitation centres. I also require a lot of assistance when my wife and child are not present, as it is becoming increasingly difficult for me to perform basic self-care tasks. On weekends and at other times when my wife is at home, she would be able to help with the care required by other residents, in addition to taking care of my needs.

I hope you will have the space available to accommodate my needs. I can be reached at ***-**** between the hours of 9 a.m. and 10 p.m. I look forward to discussing these issues with you.

Sincerely,

Sample Letter #2
This letter informs an employer that you would like to meet with him to discuss making alterations to your workplace and work schedule to accommodate your disability. This can be modified depending on your needs and the person to whom you are writing (i.e., landlord, community volunteer, minister, etc.).

Dear Bank Manager:
As you know I have been working at the bank for the last eleven years and my record has been more than satisfactory. I will be able to return to work within the next month, but as we discussed several weeks ago, several changes will have to be made before I can resume my employment.

As a result of the car accident, I use a wheelchair extensively, although I have some mobility. I will be able to perform all of my duties as deputy loan manager, as well as most of my teller duties, if these changes are made:

- the furniture is rearranged to allow a clear path for my wheelchair throughout the bank;

- the permanent chair is removed from in front of my teller window so I can work from my wheelchair;
- I am permitted to use the executive elevator and executive washroom, as the facilities on the main floor are not wheelchair accessible.

I have every confidence that these changes can be implemented swiftly. If there are any difficulties or alternatives you would like to suggest, please give me a call at ***-**** and I will be happy to discuss them. I look forward to working with you again soon.

Sincerely,

Sample Letter #3

This letter to a service club requests volunteer assistance. It can be modified depending on the group you are approaching and the topic of your request.

Dear Sir or Madam:

My name is ____ _____, and I have been diagnosed with bone cancer. It is absolutely necessary for me to receive a bone-marrow transplant in order to survive. I can receive a transplant only from someone with the same characteristics as me, and this person will be difficult to find. Finding a suitable donor is an extremely time-consuming and expensive process. I understand that your club has provided a similar service to others in my situation in the past, and I am writing to request the assistance of your organization in conducting my search for a donor.

If your organization can help me, I would be very grateful. Please give me a call at ***-**** to discuss the project. I hope to hear from you soon.

Sincerely,

Sample Letter #4
This letter to a social-service agency requests family counselling.

Dear Sir or Madam:
My husband was recently diagnosed with muscular sclerosis. In addition to all of the physical difficulties MS has caused him, he has been extremely upset since the diagnosis. His anger has been focused on me and our three children.

I love John very much, but it will be impossible to continue our relationship under the present conditions. We require effective intervention as soon as possible. I want to reinforce the strength of our marriage and ensure our family's life together.

I appreciate how hard it is for my husband to cope with this situation, but as you are aware, there are also severe difficulties for me and my children. At this point in time, my husband is not interested in marital and family counselling, but I feel that it is absolutely crucial for us to have professional intervention. Please contact me as soon as possible at ***-****. Thank you for your time.

Sincerely,

Sample Letter #5
This letter to a social-service agency requests information about support resources.

Dear Sir or Madam:
I was diagnosed with ALS several weeks ago. Needless to say, this is a very difficult time for me. My friends and family have provided me with a lot of support, but we realize that if we have to face this without outside help, it will be a very expensive and emotionally taxing situation.

I would like to contact other individuals and organizations who are experts in dealing with ALS. As far as I am aware, there is no ALS support group in our town. Do you know of anyone living in the area who has expertise in living or working with ALS? Could you also please put me in touch with the nearest regional support group? Finally, I would like to learn which facilities may be able to provide the comprehensive assistance that my family and I will require.

Please contact me at ***-****. I look forward to speaking to you soon.

Sincerely,

Sample Letter #6
This letter to a medical clinic requests an evaluation.

Dear Dr.:
My wife has recently experienced periodic episodes of blurred vision and loss of feeling in her fingers and toes. She also has experienced high-blood pressure, and last year she lost her third child in the seventh month of her pregnancy. Our family physician has indicated that these problems may be related, but at this time we do not have a firm diagnosis.

Our GP referred us to your clinic, and my wife would like to undergo a complete medical evaluation. We would like to schedule it at the earliest possible date. Enclosed are copies of my wife's medical reports. Please contact us at the number listed above. Thank you for your consideration,

Sincerely,

Sample Letter #7

This letter to a support group requests membership details and other information.

Dear Sir or Madam:

My name is ___ ____ , and I have recently been diagnosed with chronic manic depression. I am contacting you on the advice of my physician, who informed me that you and your organization would be able to provide me with information about my condition. I understand that the group also provides emotional support, and I hope to benefit from the experiences of your members, who have faced similar problems in the past.

I would like to come to one of your meetings to find out more about what you have to offer. I find it very difficult to meet people and function in social settings, and I hope your organization can help. I hope to hear from you soon.

Sincerely,

Sample Letter #8

This letter to a computer company requests information on assistive technology.

Dear Sir or Madam:

I recently read an article about your company in the newspaper. The article described a computer that is operated completely by voice. I do not have the use of my arms and hands, and this technology would open up a whole new world of possibilities for me. I have also heard that in the past, your company has provided special discounts to people with disabilities.

I would like to meet with you, or a representative of your

company, to see if this technology meets my needs. Please give me a call at ***-****. I hope to hear from you soon.

Sincerely,

Sample Letter #9

This letter to an insurance company requests early access to life insurance funds during a terminal illness. A copy of this letter should be sent to your lawyer or the agent exercising a power of attorney on your behalf. Follow your letter with a phone call if you get no response. If the insurance company is unreceptive, you should have your legal representative pursue your request.

Dear Sir or Madam:

I have been a client of your company for the last twenty-five years, and during that time your firm has provided me with comprehensive life insurance, as well as all of the other policies I have required.

Three years ago I was diagnosed with scleroderma, a degenerative disease that attacks the connective tissues of the body. This is a terminal condition. I have already lost two fingers on my right hand and the ends of four of my fingers on the left. Two of the toes on my right foot will be amputated next week.

I have reached the point where I am no longer able to pursue my career as a lawyer. The constant medication and medical care I require are extraordinarily expensive. My disability insurance is insufficient to pay for all of my needs.

As a result, I would like to request access to a portion of my life-insurance benefits while I am still alive. Other insurance companies have adopted similar payment policies, and I am asking your company to do the same. Without access to these funds, my family and I will be in dire straits, and we may be exposed to bankruptcy. As my family members will be the eventual beneficiaries of my policy, I would like to meet with you to discuss a payment plan that will address our current needs. Please contact me at the above address.

Sincerely,

Sample Letter #10

This letter to the Workers' Compensation Board informs them of a disability and requests disability benefits. It should be tailored to the specific details of your injury and claim. This letter should be crafted in consultation with your legal representative.

Dear Sir or Madam:

I have been a construction worker for the city of _____ for the past eighteen years. During that time, I operated a jackhammer as a regular part of my job with the roads department. Last week, my doctors informed me that I could no longer continue my duties because of severe damage to my kidneys. The constant vibration of the jackhammers has caused a series of ruptures, and if any further damage occurs, I risk permanent kidney failure. I therefore request that a fair settlement be negotiated under the terms of the Workers' Compensation Agreement.

I have enclosed copies of all relevant medical reports, and I am happy to be examined by any of your physicians. I would like to schedule my hearing as early as possible. Thank you for your consideration.

Sincerely,

Sample Letter #11

This letter to a travel company requests accommodation.

Dear Sir or Madam:

I have spina bifida and use a wheelchair. I would like to take my family for a vacation in the Caribbean at a resort with facilities that are fully wheelchair accessible. I live a very active life. I swim, lift weights, and play numerous wheelchair sports. I have been informed that many travel agencies have available, or are willing to design, custom vacations for people with disabilities.

At the resort, we would like to be able to take advantage of a wheelchair-accessible beach with numerous organized water sports, restaurants, theatres, and night clubs. We would also like to have access to babysitting facilities. Please give me a call at ***-****. I look forward to speaking to you soon.

Sincerely,

Sample Letter #12

This letter to a university or community college requests special-education provisions that take your disability into account.

Dear Sir or Madam:

I would like to meet with a career counsellor at your school to discuss work-training possibilities for senior students. I am forty-two years old, and an ex-police officer who was forced to take early retirement because of the effects of post-traumatic stress syndrome.

I understand your institution offers career counselling and retraining that can lead to new work. I would like to explain my condition to you so that you can offer me the most appropriate alternatives. I have a great deal of difficulty handling stress, and I can function only during daylight hours. I am computer literate, and I speak French and German, in addition to English. I am contemplating the possibility of working with juveniles in a counselling capacity. At police college, I was fourth in my class of 150, and I believe I have the potential to excel in a new career. Because of my disability, I may not be able to take a full course load, so I would be particularly interested in your options for part-time students.

I hope we can arrange a meeting within the next couple of weeks. Thank you.

Sincerely,

Sample Letter #13

This letter to a potential employer informs her of your intention to apply for a job. It also clearly explains the existence of and impact of your disability, so your employer will not be misinformed about the nature of your condition.

Dear Sir or Madam:

I would like to apply for the position of _____ in your firm. Enclosed please find my resumé, which details my educational background and work experience.

There is one detail of which I would like to make you aware. I have diabetes, which was diagnosed more than eleven years ago. The condition did not in any way affect my academic career, and it will not in any way affect my ability to carry out my job responsibilities. I am otherwise in excellent physical condition.

I believe I have all of the qualifications that are necessary for the advertised position. I hope you will provide me with fair consideration for the job, and I would welcome the opportunity to work with you. Please contact me at the above address.

Sincerely,

Sample Letter #14

This letter to your insurance lawyer informs her that you have experienced a disability that has prevented you from working, and that you would like her to proceed with a claim on your behalf.

Dear Ms. Carpenter:

On March 23, I was diagnosed with rheumatoid arthritis. Although it is in its initial stage, I know that I will not be able to continue in my job as a truck driver. I would like to meet with you and your disability assessor to determine the short- and long-term implications of my disability.

As soon as this has been done, I would like you to forward my claim to the Good News Insurance Agency, with whom I am insured. I would also like you to handle all of my negotiations with the insurance company. Please keep me informed of all developments.

Sincerely,

Appendix B

Directory of Disability-Related Organizations
Serving Persons with Disabilities

UNITED STATES

Academy of Dentistry for Persons with Disabilities
211 E. Chicago Ave.
Chicago, IL 60611
(312) 440-2661

Adventures in Movement for the Handicapped
945 Danbury Rd.
Dayton, OH 45240
(937) 294-4611
Fax: (937) 294-3783
Toll-Free: (800) 332-8210
Web site: www.AIMkids@aol.com

Advocacy Institute
1707 L St. NW, Ste. 400
Washington, DC 20036
(202) 659-8475
Fax: (202) 659-8484
E-mail: info@advocacy.org
Web site: http://advocacy.org

Alexander Graham Bell Association for the Deaf
3417 Volta Place, NW
Washington, D.C. 20007-2778
(202) 337-5220
E-mail: agbell2@aol.com
Web site: www.agbell.org

Alzheimer's Disease and Related Disorders Inc.
919 North Michigan Ave., Ste. 1000
Chicago, IL 60611-1676
(312) 335-8700
Fax: (312) 335-1110
Toll-Free: (800) 272-3900
Web site: www.alz.org

American Academy of Allergy, Asthma and Immunology (AAAAI)
611 E. Wells St.
Milwaukee, Wisconsin 53202
(414) 272-6071
Fax: (414) 276-3349
Toll-Free: (800) 822-2762

American Anorexia/Bulimia Association
165 West 45th St., Ste. 1108
New York, NY 10036
(212) 575-6200

American Association on Mental Retardation
444 N. Capitol St. NW, Ste. 846
Washington, DC 20001-1512
(202) 387-1968
Fax: (202) 387-2193
Toll-Free: (800) 424-3688
E-mail: aamr@access.digex.net
Web site: www.aamr.org

American Cancer Society
1599 Clifton Road, NE
Atlanta, GA 30329
(404) 320-3333 or (404) 329-7648
Toll-Free: (800) 227-2345
Fax: (404) 325-0230
Web site: www.cancer.org

American Civil Liberties Union
125 Broad St., 18th Fl.
New York, NY 10004
(212) 549-2500
Fax: (212) 549-2646
Toll-Free: (800) 775-2258
E-mail: aclunatl@aclu.org
Web site: www.aclu.org

American Council of the Blind
1155 15th St. NW, Ste. 720
Washington, DC 20005
(202) 467-5081
Fax: (202) 467-5085
Toll-Free: (800) 424-8666
E-mail: ncrabb@acb.org
Web site: www.acb.org

American Counseling Association
5999 Stevenson Ave.
Alexandria, VA 22304-3300
(703) 823-9800
Fax: (703) 823-0252
Toll-Free: (800) 347-6647
Web site: http://counseling.org

American Diabetes Association
P.O. Box 25757
National Center, 1660 Duke St.
Alexandria, VA 22314
(703) 549-1500
Fax: (703) 836-7439
Toll-Free: (800) 232-3472
Web site: www.diabetes.org

Americans with Disabilities Act
10765 SW 104 St.
Miami, FL 33176
(305) 271-0012 or (305) 271-0011
Fax: (305) 273-1221
E-mail: ergobobl@aol.com

American Disability Association
2201 6th Ave. S.
Birmingham, AL 35233
(205) 323-3030
Fax: (205) 251-7417
E-mail: wjf@bellsouth@net
Web site: www.adanet.org

American Foundation for the Blind
(AFB) Information Line
11 Penn Plaza, Ste. 300
New York, NY 10001
(212) 502-7600
Fax: (212) 502-7777
Toll-Free: (800) 232-5463
E-mail: NEWYORK@AFB.NET
Web site: www.afb.org

American Genetic Association
P.O. Box 257
Buckeystown, MD 21717-0257
(301) 695-9292
Fax: (301) 695-9292
E-mail: agajoh@mail.ncifcrf.gov
Web site: www.oup-usa.org

American Heart Association
7272 Greenville Ave.
Dallas, TX 75231-4596
(214) 373-6300
Fax: (214) 706-1341
Toll-Free: (800) 242-8721
E-mail: inquire@heart.org
Web site: www.americanheart.org

American Kidney Association
Toll-Free: (800) 822-4685

American Kidney Fund
6110 Executive Blvd. Ste. 1010
Rockville, MD 20852
(301) 881-3052
Fax: (301) 881-0898
Toll-Free: (800) 638-8299
E-mail: helpline@akfinc.org
Web site: www.akfinc.org

American Liver Foundation and
Hepatitis Hotline
75 Maiden Lane, Ste. 603
New York, NY 10038
(212) 668-1000
Toll-Free: (800) 223-0179
E-mail: Webmail@liverfoundation.org

American Lung Association
1740 Broadway
New York, NY 10019
(212) 315-8700
Fax: (212) 265-5642
Toll-Free: (800) 318-5864

American Network of Community
Options and Resources
4200 Evergreen Ln., Ste. 315
Annadale, VA 22003
(703) 642-6614
Fax: (703) 642-0497
E-mail: ancor@radix.net
Web site: www.ancor.org

American Occupational Therapy
Association (AOTA)
4720 Montgomery Ln.
P.O. Box 31220
Bethesda, MD 20824-1220
(301) 652-2682
Fax: (301) 652-7711
Web site: www.aota.org

American Pain Society
4700 W. Lake Ave.
Glenview, IL 60025
(847) 375-4715
Fax: (847) 975-4777
E-mail: info@ampainsoc.org
Web site: www.ampainsoc.org

American Paralyisis Association
500 Morris Ave.
Springfield, NJ 07081
(973) 379-2690
Fax: (973) 912-9433
Toll-Free: (800) 225-0292
E-mail: paralysis@aol.com
Web site: www.apacure.org

American Physical Therapy Association
111 N. Fairfax Street
Alexandria, VA 22314
(703) 683-6748
Fax: (703) 684-7343
Web site: www.apta.org

American Printing House for the Blind
1839 Frankfort Ave.
P.O. Box 6085
Louisville, KY 40206
(502) 895-2405
Fax: (502) 899-2274
Toll-Free: (800) 223-1839
E-mail: info@aph.org
Web site: www.aph.org

American Speech–Language–Hearing
Association
10801 Rockville Pike
Rockville, MD 20852
(301) 897-8682
Fax: (301) 571-0457
Toll-Free: (800) 638-8255
(Action Center)
E-mail: actioncenter@asha.org
Web site: www.asha.org

Arthritis Foundation
1330 W. Peachtree St.
Atlanta, GA 30309
(404) 872-7100
Fax: (404) 872-0457
Toll-Free: (800) 283-7800
E-mail: help@arthritis.org
Web site: www.arthritis.org

Assistance Dogs of America
8806 State Rte. 64
Swanton, OH 43558
(419) 825-3622
Fax: (419) 825-3710
E-mail: ADAIfacili@aol.com
Web site: www.adai.org

Assisted Living Facilities Association
of America
10300 Eaton Place, Ste. 400
Fairfax, VA 22030
(703) 691-8100
Fax: (703) 691-8106
Web site: www.alfa.org

Association on Higher Education
and Disability
P.O. Box 21192
Columbus, OH 43221-0192
(614) 488-4972
Fax: (614) 488-1174
E-mail: ahead@postbox.acs.ohio-state.edu
Web site: www.ahead.org

The ARC: Association for Retarded
Citizens of the United States
500 E. Border St., Ste. 300
Arlington, TX 76010
(817) 261-6003
Fax: (817) 277-3491
TDD: (817) 277-0553
Toll-Free: (800) 433-5255

Asthma and Allergy Foundation
of America
1135 15th St. NW Ste. 502
Washington, DC 20005
(202) 466-7643
Fax: (202) 466-8940
Toll-Free: (800) 727-8462
E-mail: info@aafa.org
Web site: www.aafa.org

Autism Society of America
7910 Woodmont Ave., Ste. 300
Bethesda, MD 20814
(301) 657-0881
Fax: (301) 657-0869
Toll-Free: (800) 328-8476
Web site: www.autism_ society.org/

Brain Injury Association, Inc.
105 N. Alfred
Alexandria, VA 22314
(703) 236-6000
Fax: (703) 236-6001
Toll-Free: (800) 444-6443
Web site: www.biausa.org

Cancer Care Inc.
Toll-Free: (800) 813-4673
E-mail: info@cancercare.org
Web site: www.cancercare.org

Canine Companions for Independence
P.O. Box 446
Santa Rosa, CA 95402
(707) 577-1700
Fax: (707) 577-1711
Toll-Free: (800) 572-2275
Web site: www.caninecom panions.org

CDC National Prevention Information
Network
P.O. Box 6003
Rockville, MD 20849-6003
Toll-Free: (800) 458-5231
Fax: 888-282-7681
E-mail: info@cdcnpin.org
Web site: www.cdcnpin.org

Center on Human Policy, Syracuse
University
805 S. Crouse Ave.
Syracuse, NY 13244-2280
(315) 443-3851
Fax: (315) 443-4338
Toll-Free: (800) 894-0826
Web site: soeweb.syr.edu/thechp/

Center for Law and Education
197 Friend St., 9th Fl.
Boston, MA 02114-1802
(617) 371-1166
Fax: (617) 371-1155
Web site: www.cleweb.org

Clearinghouse on Disability
Information
United States Department of Education
Office of Special Education and
Rehabilitative Services (OSERS)
330C Street SW, Rm. 3132
Washington, DC 20202-2524
(202) 205-8241
Fax: (202) 401-2608
Web site: www.ed.gov/OFFICES/OSERS

Commission on Mental and Physical
Disability Law
c/o American Bar Association
740 15th St. N.W., 9th Fl.
Washington, DC 20005
(202) 662-1570
Web site: www.abanet.org/disability

Compassion International
3955 Cragwood Dr.,
Colorado Springs, CO 80910
(719) 594-9900
Fax: (719) 594-6271
Toll-Free: (800) 336-7676
Web site: www.ci.org

Cooley's Anemia Foundation
129-09 26th Ave., Ste. 203
Flushing, NY 11354
(718) 321-2873
Fax: (718) 321-3340
Toll-Free: (800) 522-7222
E-mail: ncas@aol.com
Web site: www.thalassemia.org

The Council on Quality and Leadership
for People with Disabilities
100 West Rd., Ste. 406
Towson, MD 21204
(410) 583-0060
Fax: (410) 583-0063
E-mail: council@thecouncil.org

Crohn's and Colitis Foundation of
America
386 Park Ave. S.
NewYork, NY 10016-8804
(212) 685-3440
Fax: (212) 779-4098
Toll-Free: (800) 932-2423
E-mail: info@ccfa.org
Web site: www.ccfa.org

Cystic Fibrosis Foundation
6931 Arlington Rd., No. 200
Bethesda, MD 20814
(301) 951-4422
Fax: (301) 951-6378
Toll-Free: (800) 344-4823
E-mail: info@cff.org
Web site: www.cff.org

Disability Rights Education and
Defense Fund
2212 6th St.
Berkeley, CA 94710
(510) 644-2555
Fax: (510) 841-8645
ADA Hotline: (510) 644-2626
Web site: www.dredf.org

Disabled Sports U.S.
Web site: www.dsusa.org/~
dsusa/links.h

Dystonia Medical Research Foundation
1 E. Wacker Dr., Ste. 2430
Chicago, IL 60601-1905
(312) 755-0198
Fax: (312) 803-0138
Toll-Free: (800) 377-3978

Easter Seals
230 West Monroe St., Ste. 1800
Chicago, IL 60606-4802
(312) 726-6200
TDD: (312) 726-4258
Fax: (312) 726-1494
Web site: www.easter_seals.org

Epilepsy Foundation
4351 Garden City Drive Ste. 500
Landover, MD 20785
(301) 459-3700
Fax: (301) 577-2684
Toll-Free: (800) 332-1000
E-mail: postmaster@efa.org
Web site: www.efa.org

Evan Kemp Associates, Health and Mobility
9151 Hampton Overlook
Capitol Heights, MD 20743
(301) 324-0112

Federal Employment and Guidance Service
114 5th Ave., 11th Fl.
New York, NY 10011
(212) 366-8400 or (516) 496-7550
Fax: (212) 366-8490
Web site: www.fegs.org

Flying Wheels Travel
143 West Bridge
P.O. Box 382
Owatonna, MN 55060
Toll Free: (800) 535-6790
Web site: www.flyingwheels.com

Goodwill Industries International Inc.
9200 Rockville Pike
Bethesda MD 20814
(301) 530-6500
Fax: (301) 530-1516
TDD: (301) 530-9579
Web site: www.goodwill.org

Guide Dogs of America
13445 Glenoaks Blvd.
Sylmar, CA 91342
(818) 362-5834
Fax: (818) 362-6870
Toll-Free: (800) 459-4843

Guide Dogs for the Blind
P.O. Box 151200
San Rafael, CA 94915-1200
(415) 499-4000
Fax: (415) 499-4035
Toll-Free: (800) 295-4050
Web site: www.guidedogs.com

Guiding Eyes for the Blind
611 Granite Springs Rd.
Yorktown Heights, NY 10598
(914) 245-4024
Fax: (914) 245-1609
Toll-Free: (800)942-0149
TDD: (800) 421-1200
E-mail: info@guiding-eyes.org
Web site: info@guiding-eyes.org

Hear Now
9745 E. Hampden Ave., Ste.300
Denver, CO 80231
(303) 695-7797
Fax: (303) 695-7789
TDD/Toll-Free: (800) 648-4327
Web site: www.leisurelan.com\~hearnow\

Helen Keller International
90 Washington St., 15th Fl.
New York, NY 10006
(212) 943-0890
Fax: (212) 943-1220
Web site: www.hki.org/

Hemophilia Resources of America Inc.
387 Pasaic Ave.
Fairfield, NJ 07004
(973) 882-8777
Fax: (973) 882-1696
Toll-Free: (800) 549-2654

Huntington's Disease Society of America, Inc.
158 West 29th-7th Fl.
New York, NY 10001
(212) 242-1968
Fax: (212) 239-3430
Toll-Free: (800) 345-4372
Web site: hdsa.mgh.harvard.edu

Independent Educational Consultants Association
4085 Chain Bridge Rd., Ste. 401
Fairfax, VA 22030-4106
(703) 591-4850
Toll-Free: (800) 808-4322
www.educationalconsulting.org

Industry-Labor Council National Center for Disability Services
201 I.U. Willets Rd.
Albertson, NY 11507-1599
(516) 747-6323
Fax: (516) 747-2046
Web site: www.business-disability.com

International Association of Official Human Rights Advocates
444 N. Capitol St., Ste. 408
Washington, DC 20001
(202) 624-5410

International Association for the Study of Pain
909 N.E. 43rd Street, Suite 306
Seattle, WA 98105-6020
(206) 547-6409
Fax: (206) 547-1703
Web site: www.halycon.com/iasp

International Hearing Society Hearing Aid Help-Line
16880 Middlebelt Rd.
Livonia, MI 48152
(734) 522-7200
Fax: (734) 533-0200
Toll-Free: (800) 521-5247
Web site: www.hearingihs.org

International Rett Syndrome Association
9121 Piscataway Rd., No. 2B
Clinton, MD 20735
(301) 856-3334
Fax: (301) 856-3336
Toll-Free: (800) 818-7388
Web site: www.rettsyndrome.org

Learning Disabilities Association of America
4156 Library Rd.
Pittsburgh, PA 15234
(412) 341-1515
Fax: (412) 344-0224
Toll-Free: (888) 300-6710
E-mail: ldnatl@vsaor.net
Web site: www.ldanatl.org

Leukemia Society of America
600 Third Ave.
New York, NY 10016
(212) 573-8484
Fax: (212) 856-9686
Toll-Free: (800) 955-4572
Web site: www.leukemia.org/docs/lsa2.s

Mainstream
3 Bethesda Metro Center, Ste. 830
Bethesda, MD 20814
(301) 654-2400
Fax: (301) 654-2403
TDD: (202) 654-2400
Web site: www.mainstream-mag.com

March of Dimes
1275 Mamaroneck Avenue
White Plains, NY 10605
(914) 428-7100
Fax: (914) 428-8203
Toll-Free: (800) 443-4093
Web site: www.modimes.org

Medic Alert Foundation International
P.O. Box 3644
Albuquerque, NM 87190
(505) 884-3008 (24 hrs.)
http://totah.infoway.lib.nm.us/HelpLin

Muscular Dystrophy Association of America
3300 E. Sunrise Dr.
Tucson, AZ 85718
(520) 529-2000
Fax: (520) 529-5300
Toll-Free: (800) 572-1717
Web site: www.mdausa.org

Myasthenia Gravis Foundation, Inc.
225 S. Riverside Plaza, Ste. 1540
Chicago, IL 60606
(312) 258-0522
Fax: (312) 258-0461
Toll-Free: (800) 541-5454
Web site: www.myasthenia.org

National Adrenal Diseases Foundation
505 Northern Blvd. Ste. 200
Great Neck, NY 11021
(516) 487-4992
Web site: http://medhlp.netusa.net/agsg
/agsg

National AIDS Hotline
Toll-Free: (800) 342-2437 or
(800) 243-7889
Web site: www.aoa.dhhs.gov/aoa
/dir/12

National Amputation Foundation
38-40 Church St.
Malverne, NY 11565
(516) 887-3600
Fax: (516) 887-3667

**National Association of Anorexia
Nervosa and Associated Disorders**
Box 7
Highland Park, IL 60035
(847) 831-3438
Fax: (847) 433-4632
E-mail: anad20@aol.com

National Association of the Deaf
814 Thayer Avenue
Silver Spring, MD 20910-4500
(301) 587-1788
Fax: (301) 587-1791
TTY: (301) 587-1789
E-mail: nadinfo@nad.org
Web site: www.igc.apc.org\ NADDC

**National Association of Developmental
Disabilities Councils**
1234 Massachusetts Ave. NW, Ste. 103
Washington, DC 20005
(202) 347-1234
Fax: (202) 347-4023
E-mail: naddc@igc.apc.org

**National Association for Down
Syndrome**
P.O. Box 4542
Oak Brook, IL 60522-4542
(630) 325-9112

National Association for Home Care
519 C Street, N.E., Stanton Park
Washington, DC 20002
(202) 547-7424
Fax: (202) 547-3540
Web site: www.nahc.org

**National Association of Insurance
Commissioners**
120 West 12th Street, Ste. 1100
Kansas City, MO 64105-1925
(816) 842-3600
Fax: (816) 471-7004
Web site: www.naic.org

**National Association of the Physically
Handicapped**
Bethesda Scarlet Oaks, No. 6A4
440 Lafayette Ave.
Cincinnati, OH 45220-1000
(517) 799-3060
Web site: www.naph.net

**National Association of Protection and
Advocacy Systems**
900 2nd St. NE, Ste. 211
Washington, DC 20002
(202) 408-9514
Fax: (202) 408-9520
www.protectionandadvocacy.com

**National Benevolent Association of the
Christian Church**
11780 Borman Dr.,
St. Louis, MO 63146-4157
(314) 993-9000

National Center for Learning
Disabilities
381 Park Ave. S., Ste. 1401
New York, NY 10016
(212) 545-7510
Fax: (212) 545-9665
Toll-Free: (888) 575-7373
Web site: www.ncld.org

National Charities Information Bureau
19 Union Square West
New York, NY 10003
(212) 929-6300
Fax: (212) 463-7083
Toll-Free: (800) 501-6242
Web site: www.give.org

National Council on Independent
Living
1916 Wilson Blvd., Ste. 209
Arlington, VA 22201
(703) 525-3406

National Down Syndrome Congress
7000 Peachtree-Dunwoody Rd. N.E.
Bldg. 5, Ste. 100
Atlanta, GA 30328
(770) 604-9500
Fax: (770) 604-9898
Toll-Free: (800) 232-6372
Web site: www.members. carol.net/ndsc

National Down Syndrome Society
666 Broadway
New York, NY 10012
(212) 460-9330
Fax: (212) 979-2873
Toll-Free: (800) 221-4602
Web site: www.ndss.org

National Federation of the Blind
1800 Johnson Street
Baltimore, MD 21230
(410) 659-9314
Fax: (410) 685-5653
Web site: www.nfb.org

National Foundation of Dentistry for
the Handicapped
1800 15th St., Unit 100
Denver, CO 80202
(303) 534-5360
Fax: (303) 534-5290

National Foundation for Facial
Reconstruction
317 E. 34th St., Ste. 901
New York, NY 10016
(212) 263-6656
Fax: (212) 263-7534
Web site: www.nffr.org

National Foundation for Transplants
1102 Brookfield, Ste. 202
Memphis, TN 38119
(901) 684-1697
Fax: (901) 684-1128
Toll-Free: (800) 489-3863
Web site: www.transplants.org

National Hearing Dog Project
American Humane Association
63 Inverness Dr. East
Englewood, CO 80112
(303) 792-9900
Fax: (303) 792-5333
Toll-Free: (800) 227-4645
Web site: www.americanhumane.org

National Hemophilia Foundation
116 W. 32nd Street, 11th Fl.
New York, NY 10001
(212) 328-3700
Fax: (212) 328-3777
Web site: www.hemophilia.org

National Institute for Rehabilitation
Engineering
P.O. Box T
Hewitt, NJ 07421
(201) 853-6585
Fax: (800) 736-2216
E-mail: nire@theoffice.net
Web site: www.theoffice.net/nire

NISH (Employment Service)
2235 Cedar Ln.
Vienna, VA 22182-5200
(703) 560-6800
Fax: (703) 849-8916
Web site: www.nish.org

National Kidney Foundation, Inc.
30 East 33rd Street, Ste. 1100
New York, NY 10016
(212) 889-2210
Fax: (212) 689-9261
Toll-Free: (800) 622-9010
Web site: www.kidney.org

National Library Service for the Blind
and Physically Handicapped
Washington, DC 20542
Web site: www.crrl.org/services/outreac

National Marfan Foundation
382 Main Street
Port Washington, NY 11050
(516) 883-8712
Fax: (516) 883-8040
Toll-Free: (800) 862-7326
Web site: www.marfan.otg

National Mental Health Association –
Information Center
1021 Prince Street
Alexandria, VA 22314-2971
(703) 684-7722
Fax: (702) 684-5968
Toll-Free: (800) 969-6642
Web site: www.nmha.org

National Multiple Sclerosis Society
733 3rd Ave.
New York, NY 10017
(212) 986-3240
Fax: (212) 986-7981
Toll-Free: (800) 344-4867
Web site: www.nmss.org

National Neurofibramatosis
Foundation
95 Pine St., 16th Fl.
New York, NY 10005
(212) 344-6633
Fax: (212) 747-0004
Toll-Free: (800) 323-7938
Web site: www.neurofibramatosis.org

National Organization on Disability
910 16th St. NW, Ste. 600
Washington, DC 20006
(202) 293-5960
Fax: (202) 293-7999
Web site: www.nod.org

National Organization for Rare
Disorders
P.O. Box 8923
New Fairfield, CT 06812
(203) 746-6518
Fax: (203) 746-6481
Web site: www.rarediseases.org

National Rehabilitation Association
633 South Washington Street
Alexandria, VA 22314
(703) 836-0850
Fax: (703) 836-0848
Web site: www.nationalrehab.org

National Rehabilitation Counseling
Association
8807 Sudley Rd., Ste. 102
Manassas, VA 20110-4719
(703) 361-2077
Fax: (703) 361-2489
E-mail: nrcaoffice@aol.com

National Scoliosis Foundation
5 Cabot Place
Stoughton, MA 02072
(617) 341-6333
http://medhlp.netusa.net/agsg/agsg

National Self-Help Clearinghouse
25 W. 43rd St. Rm. 620
New York, NY, 10036-7406
(212) 354-8525
Fax: (212) 642-1956
Web site: www.selfhelpweb.org

National Sickle-Cell Disease Program
Division of Blood Diseases and
Resources
National Heart, Lung, and Blood
Institute
2 Rockledge Center
6701 Rockledge Drive MSC 7950
Bethesda, MD 20892-7950
(301) 435-0055
Fax: (301) 480-0868

National Spinal Cord Injury
Association
300 Colesville Rd., Ste. 551
Silver Spring MD 20910
(301) 588-6959
Fax: (301) 588-9414
Toll-Free: (800) 962-9629
Web site: www.spinalcord.org

NTID's Center on Employment
National Technical Institute for the
Deaf
Rochester Institute of Technology
52 Lomb Memorial Drive
Rochester, NY 14623-5604
(716) 475-6219
Fax: (716) 475-7570
Web site: www.rit.edu/NTID/CO/CE

National Tuberous Sclerosis Association
of America
8181 Professional Place, Ste. 110
Landover, MD 20785
(301) 459-9888
Fax: (301) 459-0394
Toll-Free: (800) 225-6872
Web site: www.ntsa.org

National Wheelchair Basketball
Association
Web site: www.nwba.org

North American Riding for the
Handicapped Association
P.O. Box 33150
Denver, CO 80233
(303) 452-1212
Fax: (303) 252-4610
Toll-Free: (800) 369-7433
Web site: www.narha.org

Paralyzed Veterans of America
801 18th Street, NW
Washington, D.C. 20006
(202) 872-1300
Fax: (202) 785-4452
Toll-Free: (800) 424-8200
Web site: www.pva.org

Parkinson's Disease Foundation
William Black Medical Research
Buliding
Columbia Presbyterian Medical Center
710 W. 168th St.
New York, NY 10032
(212) 923-4700
Fax: (212) 923-4778
Toll-Free: (800) 457-6676
www.parkinsonsfoundation.org

Partners of the Americas Rehabilitation
Education Program
1424 K St. NW, Ste. 700
Washington, DC 20005
(202) 628-3300
Fax: (202) 628-3306
Web site: www.partners.net

People-to-People Committee on
Disability
P.O. Box 18131
Washington, DC 20036
(703) 535-6011
Fax: (703) 836-0367
Web site: www.iftdo.org

Prader-Willi Syndrome Association
5700 Midnight Pass Road, Ste. 6
Sarasota, FL 34242
(941) 312-0400
Fax: (941) 312-0142
Web site: www.pwsausa.org

Project HEATH/HEATH Resource
Center
1 Dupont Cir., Ste. 800
Washington DC, 20036-1193
(202) 939-9320
Fax: (202) 833-4760
Toll-Free: (800) 544-3284
Web site: www.acenet.edu

Rehabilitation Engineering and
Assistive Technology Society of North
America
1700 N. Moore St., Ste. 1540
Arlington, VA 22209-1903
(703) 524-6686
Fax: (703) 524-6630
Web site: www.resna.org

Rehabilitation International
25 East 21st Street
New York, NY 10010
(212) 420-1500
Fax: (212) 505-0871
Web site: www.rehabintl.org

Self-Help for Hard of Hearing People
7910 Woodmont Ave., Ste. 1200
Bethesda, MD 20814
(301) 657-2248
Fax: (301) 913-9413
Web site: www.shhh.org

Sexuality Information Education
Council of the United States
130 W. 42nd St., Ste. 350
New York, NY 10036
(212) 819-9770
Fax: (212) 819-9776
Web site: http://siecus.org

Society for the Advancement of
Travellers with Handicaps
347 5th Ave., Ste. 610
New York, NY 10016
(212) 447-7284
Fax: (212) 725-8253

Special Olympics, Inc.
1325 G St. NW, Ste. 500
Washington, DC 20005
(202) 628-3630
Fax: (202) 824-0200
Toll-Free: (800) 700-8585
Web site: www.specialolympics.org

Spina Bifida Association of America
4590 MacArthur Blvd. NW, Ste. 250
Washington, DC 20007-4226
(202) 944-3295
Fax: (202) 944-3295
Toll-Free: (800) 621-3141
Web site: www.sbaa.org

STD National Hotline (C.D.C.
National S.T.D. Hotline)
Toll-Free: (800) 227-8922
Web site: http://ashastd.org/std/stdhotln

Sports A to Z: Disabled Sports
Web site: www.olympic.usa.org/sports/a

Symbral Foundation (Financial
Assistance)
7826 Eastern Ave. NW, Ste. 18A, LL18
Washington, DC 20012
(202) 726-1444
Fax: (202) 726-1448

TASH (Support Group)
29 W. Susquehanna Ave., Ste. 210
Baltimore, MD 21204
(410) 828-8274
Toll-Free: (800) 482-8274
Web site: www.tash.org

Thyroid Foundation of America
Ruth Sleeper Hall, RSL 350
40 Parkman St.
Boston, MA 02114
(617) 726-8500
Fax: (617) 726-4136
Toll-Free: (800) 832-8321
Web site: www.clark.net/pub/tfa

Tourette Syndrome Association
42-40 Bell Blvd., Ste. 205
Bayside, NY 11361
(718) 224-2999
Fax: (718) 279-9596
Toll-Free: (800) 237-0717
Web site: http://tsa.mgh.harvard.edu/

Transplant Recipients International Organization
1000 16th St. NW Ste. 602
Washington, DC 20036-5705
(202) 293-0980
Fax: (202) 293-0973
Toll-Free: (800) 876-3386
Web site: http://trioweb.org

Turner Syndrome Society of the United States
1313 S.E. 5th St. Ste. 327
Minneapolis, MN 55414
(612) 379-3607
Fax: (612) 379-3619
Toll-Free: (800) 365-9944
Web site: www.turner-syndrome-us.org

United Cerebral Palsy Association
1660 L St. NW, Ste. 700
Washington, DC 20036
(202) 776-0406
Toll-Free: (800) 872-5827
Web site: www.ucpa.org

United Ostomy Association
19772 MacArthur Blvd., Ste. 200
Irvine, CA 92612
(949) 660-8624
Fax: (949) 660-9262
Toll-Free: (800) 826-0826
Web site: www.uoa.org

United States Cerebral Palsy Athletic Association
200 Harrison Ave.
Newport, RI 02840
(410) 848-2460
Fax: (401) 848-5280
Web site: www.uscpaa.org

Very Special Arts
John F. Kennedy Center for the
Performing Arts Education Office
Washington, DC 20566
(202) 628-2800
Fax: (202) 737-0725
Toll-Free: (800) 933-8721
Web site: www.vsarts.org

Voice of the Retarded
5005 Newport Dr., Ste. 108
Rolling Meadows, IL 60008
(847) 253-6020
Fax: (847) 253-6054
E-mail: vor@compuserve.com

Volunteers of America—National Office
110 South Union St.
Alexandria, VA 22314-3324
Fax: (703) 684-1972
Toll-Free: (800) 899-0089
Web site: www.voa.org

Wheelchair Sports, USA
3595 E. Fountain Blvd., Ste. L-1
Colorado Springs, CO 80910
(719) 574-1150
Fax: (719) 574-9840
Web site: www.wsusa.org

World Institute on Disability
510 16th St., Ste. 100
Oakland, CA 94612
(510) 763-4100
Fax: (510) 763-4109
Web site: www.wid.org

CANADA

Ability Online Support Network
919 Alness St.
North York ON M3J 2J1
(416) 650-6207
Fax: (416) 650-5073
Modem: (416) 650-5411
E-mail: info@ablelink.org
Web site: www.ablelink.org

AboutFace
123 Edward St., Suite 1003
Toronto, ON M5G 1E2
(416) 997-2229
Fax: (416) 597-8494
Toll-Free: (800) 665-3223

Accessible Transportation Directorate
c/o Canadian Transportation Agency
15 Eddy St.
Hull, QC K1A 0N9
(819) 997-6828
Fax: (819) 953-6019
Toll-Free: (800) 883-1813
TTY: (800) 669-5575
Web site: www.cta-otc.gc.ca

Acoustic Neuroma Association of Canada (ANAC)
P.O. Box 369
Edmonton, AB T5J 2J6
(403) 428-3384
Fax: (403) 425-8519
Toll-Free: (800) 561-2622
E-mail: anac@compusmart.ab.ca

Active Living Alliance for Canadians with a Disability
1101 Prince of Wales Dr., Suite 230
Ottawa, ON K2C 3W7
(613) 723-8710
Fax: (613) 723-1060
Toll-Free: (800) 771-0663
disability.alliance@activeliving.ca
www.activeliving.ca/activeliving/alliance/alliance.html

Adaptive Technology Resource Centre (ATRC)
c/o J.P. Robarts Library
University of Toronto
130 St. George St., 1st floor
Toronto, ON M5S 2T4
(416) 946-3225
Fax: (416) 971-2629
E-mail: general.atrc@utoronto.ca
Web site: www.utoronto.ca/atrc

Allergy and Asthma Information Association of Canada
30 Eglinton Ave. W., Suite 750
Mississauga, ON L5R 3E7
(905) 712-2242
Fax: (905) 712-2245
Toll-Free: (800) 611-7011

ALS Society of Canada
6 Adelaide St. E., Suite 220
Toronto, ON M5C 1H6
(416) 362-0269
Fax: (416) 362-0414
Toll-Free: (800) 267-4257
E-mail: alssoc@inforamp.net
Web site: www.als.ca

Alzheimer Society of Canada/Societe Alzheimer du Canada
20 Eglinton Ave. W., Suite 1200
Toronto, ON M4R 1K8
(416) 488-8772
Fax: (416) 488-3778
Toll-Free: (800) 616-8816
E-mail: info@alzheimer.ca
Web site: www.alzheimer.ca

ARCH: A Legal Resource Centre for Persons with Disabilities
40 Orchard View Blvd. Ste. 255
Toronto, ON M4R 1B9
(416) 482-8255
Fax: (416) 482-2981
TDD: (416) 482-1254
E-mail: archlawl@fox.nstn.ca
Web site: www.indie.ca/arch

L'ARCHE Canada
6646 Monk Blvd.
Montreal, QC H4E 3J1
(514) 768-5422
Fax: 514-761-0823
E-mail: jcp@sympatico.ca

The Arthritis Society – National Division
1700–393 University Ave.
Toronto, ON M5G 1E6
(416) 979-7228
Fax: (416) 979-8366
E-mail: dmorrice@arthritis.ca
Web site: www.arthritis.ca

Association for the Neurologically Disabled of Canada
59 Clement Rd.
Etobicoke, ON M9R 1Y5
(416) 244-1992
Fax: (416) 244-4099
Toll-Free: (800) 561-1497
E-mail: info@and.ca
Web site: www.and.ca

Asthma Society of Canada
425–130 Bridgeland Ave.
Toronto, ON M6A 1Z4
(416) 787-4050
Fax: (416) 787-5807
Toll-Free: (800) 787-3880
Web site: www.asthmasociety.com

Audio Vision Canada
150 Laird Dr. Annex Bldg.
Toronto, ON M4G 3V7
(416) 422-4222
Fax: (416) 422-1633
Toll-Free: (800) 567-6755
E-mail: nbrs@idirect.com
http://webhome.idirect.com/~nbrs

Autism Society of Canada
130 Bridgeland Ave., Suite 425
North York, ON M6A 1Z4
(416) 922-0302
Fax: (416) 922-1032

Back Association of Canada
80 Collingham St.
Toronto, ON M4V 1B9
(416) 967-4670

Canada Mortgage and Housing Corporation (CMHC) – National Office (Meeting Special Needs)
700 Montreal Rd.
Ottawa, ON K1A 0P7
(613) 748-2000
Fax: (613) 748-2098
E-mail: chic@cmhc-schl.gc.ca
Web site: www.cmhc.ca/cmhc.html

Canada Pension Plan – CPP
Toll-Free: (800) 277-9914
Toll-Free: (800) 277-9915 (French)
TTY: (800) 255-4787
Web site: www.htdc.gc.ca/isp

Canadian Abilities Foundation
501–489 College St.
Toronto, ON M6G 1A5
(416) 923-1885
Fax: 416-923-9829
E-mail: able@interlog.com
Web site: http://indie.ca/abilities/

Canadian AIDS Society
900–130 Albert St.
Ottawa, ON K1P 5G4
(613) 230-3580
Fax: (613) 563-4998
Toll-Free: (800) 884-1058
E-mail: casinfo@cdnaids.ca
Web site: www.cdnids.ca

Canadian Amputee Sports Association (CASA)
428 Lake Bonavista Dr. SE
Calgary, AB T2J 0M1
(403) 278-8772
Fax: (403) 271-1920

Canadian Association for
Community Living
c/o York University
Kinsmen Building
4700 Keele St.
North York, ON M3J 1P3
(416) 661-9611
Fax: (416) 661-5701
TTY: (416) 661-2023
Toll Free: (800) 856-2207
E-mail: info@cacl.ca
Web site: www.cacl.ca

Canadian Association of the Deaf
251 Bank St., Suite 203
Ottawa, ON K2P 1X3
(613) 565-2882
Fax: (613) 565-1207
TTY: (613) 565-2882
Web site: www.cad.ca

Canadian Association of Independent
Living Centres (CAILC)
1004–350 Sparks St.
Ottawa, ON K1R 7S8
(613) 563-2581
Fax: (613) 235-4497
TTY: (613) 563-2581
Web site: http://indie.htm

Canadian Association of Occupational
Therapists (CAOT)
Carleton Technology and Training
Center
1125 Colonel By Drive, Suite 3400
Ottawa, ON K1S 5R1
(613) 523-2268
Fax: (613) 523-2552
Web site: www.caot.ca

Canadian Association of Rehabilitation
Professionals (CARP)
500-7030 Woodbine Ave.
Markham, ON L3R 6G2
(905) 940-9156
Fax: (905) 940-8496
Toll-Free: (888) 876-9922

Canadian Association for Research in
Rehabilitation (CARR) Canadian
Journal of Rehabilitation
c/o Rick Hansen Centre
University of Alberta
WI – 67, Van Vliet Centre
Edmonton AB T6G 2H9
(780) 492-1734
Fax: (780) 492-1626

Canadian Association of Speech-
Language Pathologists and Audiologists
2006-130 Albert St.
Ottawa, ON K1P 5G4
(613) 567-9968
Fax: (613) 567- 2859
Toll-Free: (800) 259-8519
E-mail: caslpa@caslpa.ca
Web site: www.caslpa.ca

Canadian Brain Injury Coalition
29 Pearce Avenue
Winnipeg, MB R2V 2K3
(204) 334-0471
Fax: (204) 339-1034
Toll-Free: (800) 735-2242
Web site: www.cbic.ca

Canadian Cancer Society
10 Alcorn Ave., Suite 200
Toronto, ON M4V 3B1
(416) 961-7223
Fax: (416) 961-4189
Web site: www.cancer.ca

Canadian Celiac Association – National
Office
190 Britannia Rd. E., Unit 11
Mississauga, ON L47 1W6
(905) 507-6208
Fax: (905) 507-4673
Toll-Free: (800) 363-7296
Web site: www.celiac.ca

APPENDIX B

Canadian Centre for Philanthropy
1329 Bay St., 2nd floor
Toronto, ON M5R 2C4
(416) 515-0764
Fax: (416) 515-0773
Toll-Free: (800) 263-1178
E-mail: ccp@ccp.ca
Web site: www.web.net/imagine/

Canadian Centre on Disability Studies
(CCDS)
2404-7 Evergreen Place
Winnipeg, MB R3L 2T3
(204) 287-8411
Fax: (204) 284-5343
E-mail: ccds@escape.ca
Web site: www.escape.ca/ccds/

Canadian Clearing House on Disability
Issues
c/o Office for Disability Issues
Human Resources Development
Canada
100-25 Eddy St.
Hull, QC K1A 0M5
(819) 994-7514
Fax: (819) 953-4797
Toll-Free: (800) 665-9017
TTY: (800) 561-9706

Canadian Council of the Blind
200-396 Cooper St.
Ottawa, ON K2P 2H7
(613) 567-0311
Fax: (613) 567-2728

Canadian Council on Rehabilitation
and Work (CCRW)
500 University Ave., Suite 302
Toronto, ON M5G 1V7
(416) 260-3060
Fax: (416) 260-3093
TTY: (416) 260-9223
E-mail: info@ccrw.org
Web site: www.workink.com

Canadian Cystic Fibrosis Foundation
601-2221 Yonge St.
Toronto, ON M4S 2B4
(416) 485-9149
Fax: (416) 485-0960
Toll-Free: (800) 378-2233
E-Mail: postmaster@ccff.ca
Web site: www.ccff/ca/~
cfwww/index.html

Canadian Diabetes Association
800-15 Toronto St.
Toronto, ON M5C 2E3
(416) 363-0177
Fax: (416) 363-8335
Toll-Free: (800) 226-8464
E-mail: info@diabetes.ca
Web site: www.diabetes.ca

Canadian Down Syndrome Society
811-14th St. N.W.
Calgary, AB T2N 2A4
(403) 270-8500
Fax: (403) 270-8291
Toll-Free: (800) 883-5608
E-mail: cdss@ican.net
Web site: http://home.ican.net/~
cdss/index.html

Canadian Federation of Sport
Organizations for People with
Disabilities
1600 James Naismith Dr.
Gloucester, ON
(613) 748-5630
Fax: (613) 748-5731

Canadian Foundation for Physically
Disabled Persons
731 Runnymede Rd.
Toronto, ON M6N 3V7
(416) 760-7351
Fax: (416) 760-9405
E-mail: whynot@sympatico.ca

Canadian Foundation of Genetic
Diseases Network
UBC–2125 East Mall, Rm. 249
Vancouver, BC V6T 1Z4
(604) 822-7189
Fax: (604) 822-7945
E-mail: dshindler.cgdn@ubc.ca
www.cgdn.generes.ca/index.html

Canadian Guide Dogs for the Blind
4120 Rideau Valley Dr. N.
P.O. Box 280
Manotick, ON K4M 1A3
(613) 692-7777
Fax: (613) 692-0650
E-mail: cgdb@sympatico.ca

Canadian Hard of Hearing Association
(CCHA) National Office
205-2435 Holly Lane
Ottawa, ON K1V 7P2
(613) 526-1584
Fax: (613) 526-4718
Toll-Free: (800) 263-8068
TTY 613-526-2692
E-mail: chhanational@chha.ca
Web site: www.chha.ca

Canadian Hearing Society
271 Spadina Road
Toronto, ON M5R 2V3
(416) 964-9595
Fax: (416) 928-2525
Toll-Free: (800) 465-4327
TTY: (416) 964-0023
E-mail: info@chs.ca
Web site: www.chs.ca

Canadian Hemophilia Society –
National Office
625 President Kennedy, Suite 1210
Montreal, QC H3A 1K2
(514) 848-9661
E-Mail: chs@odyssee.net

Canadian Human Rights Commission
344 Slater St., 8th Floor
Ottawa, ON K1A 1E1
(613) 995-1151
Fax: (613) 996-9661
TTY: (613) 996-5211
Toll-Free: (888) 214-1090
Toll-Free TTY: (888) 643-3304
E-mail: info.com@chrc-ccdp.ca
Web site: www.chrc-ccdp.ca

Canadian Injured Workers Alliance
P.O. Box 3678
Thunder Bay, ON P7B 6E3
(807) 345-3429
Fax: (807) 344-8683
E-mail: ciwa@norlink.net
Web site: www.ciwa.ca

Canadian Institute For Barrier Free
Design
c/o Faculty of Architecture
201 Russell Building
University of Manitoba
Winnipeg, MB R3T 2N2
(204) 474-8588
Fax: (204) 474-7532
E-mail: universal_design@umanitoba.ca

Canadian Liver Foundation
200-365 Bloor St. E.
Toronto, ON M4W 3L4
(416) 964-1953
Fax: (416) 964-0024
Toll-Free: (800) 563-5483
E-Mail: clf@liver.ca
Web site: www.liver.ca

Canadian Marfan Association (CMA)
Central Plaza Postal Outlet
128 Queen St. S., P.O. Box 42257
Mississauga, ON L5M 4Z0
(905) 826-3223
Fax: (905) 826-2125
Web site: www.marfan.ca

Canadian MedicAlert Foundation
250 Ferrand Drive, Ste. 301
Postal Station Don Mills, Box 9800
Toronto, ON M3C 2T9
(416) 696-0267
Fax: (416) 696-0156
Toll-Free: (800) 668-1507 (English)
Toll-Free: (800) 392-8422 (French)
E-mail: medicalert@flexnet.com
Web site: www.medicalert.ca

**Canadian Mental Health Association –
National Office**
2160 Yonge St., 3rd Floor
Toronto, ON M4S 2Z3
(416) 484-7750
Fax: (416) 484-4617
E-mail: cmhanat@interlog.com
Web site: www.cmha.ca

**Canadian National Home Care
Association**
(613) 569-1585
Fax: (613) 569-1604
E-mail: chca@travel-net.com
Web site: www.travel-net.com

**The Canadian National Institute for the
Blind – National Office**
1929 Bayview Ave.
Toronto, ON M4G 3E8
(416) 480-7580
Fax: (416) 480-7677
Web site: www.cnib.ca

**CNIB Information Resource Centre
(IRC)**
1929 Bayview Ave.
Toronto, ON M4G 3E8
(416) 480-7498
Fax: (416) 480-7700
Toll-Free: (800) 268-8818
E-mail: irc@lib.cnib.ca
Web site: www.cnib.ca

**Canadian Organization for Rare
Disorders (CORD)**
P.O. Box 814
Coaldale, AB T1M 1M7
(403) 345-4544
Fax: (403) 345-3948
E-mail: cord@bulli.com
Web site: www.bulli.com/~cord/

**Canadian Paraplegic Association –
National Office**
1101 Prince of Wales Drive, Suite 230
Ottawa, ON K2C 3W7
(613) 723-1033
Fax: (613) 723-1060
Web site: www.canparaplegic.org

Canadian Physiotherapy Association
2345 Yonge St., Suite 410
Toronto, ON MP4 2E5
(416) 932-1888
Fax: (416) 932-9708
Toll-Free: (800) 387-8679
E-mail: information@physiotherapy.ca
Web site: www.physiotherapy.ca

Canadian Psychiatric Association
441 MacLaren, Suite 260
Ottawa, ON K2P 2H3
(613) 234-2815
Fax: (613) 234-9857
E-mail: cpa@medical.org
Web site: http://cpa.medical.org

Canadian Public Health Association
1565 Carling Ave., Suite 400
Ottawa, ON K1Z 8R1
(613) 725-9826
Fax: (613) 725-9826
www.worldexport.com/tc98/on

Canadian Red Cross National Office
1430 Blair Place, 3rd Floor
Gloucester, ON K1J 9N2
E-mail: info@redcross.ca
Web site: http://redcross.ca

Canadian Special Olympics
40 St. Clair Ave. W., Suite 209
Toronto, ON M4V 1M2
(416) 927-9050
Fax: (416) 927-8475
E-mail: solympic@inforamp.net

Centre for Sight Enhancement
School of Optometry
University of Waterloo
Waterloo, ON N2L 3G1
(519) 888-4708
Fax: (519) 746-2337
Toll-Free: (800) 565-5965
E-mail: pbevers@sciborg.uwaterloo.ca

Centre for Studies in Aging (CSIA)
c/o Sunnybrook & Women's College
Health Sciences Centre
2075 Bayview Ave.
Toronto, ON M4N 3M5
(416) 480-5858
Fax: (416) 480-5868
csia@srcl.sunnybrook.utoronto.ca
Web site: www.sunnybrook.
utoronto.ca:8080/~csia

Council of Canadians with Disabilities
926-294 Portage Ave.
Winnipeg, MB
(204) 947-0303
E-mail: ccd@pcs.mb.ca
Web site: www.pcs.mb.ca/~ccd/

Crohn's and Colitis Foundation of
Canada (CCFC)
301-21 St. Clair Ave.E.
Toronto, ON M4T 1L9
(416) 920-5035
Fax: (416) 929-0364
Toll-Free: (800) 387-1479
E-mail: ccfc@netcom.ca
Web site: www.ccfc.ca

Disabled People's International (DPI)
101-7 Evergreen Place
Winnipeg, MB R3L 2T3
(204) 287-8010
Fax: (204) 453-1367
Toll-Free: (800) 749-7773
E-mail: d.i@dpi.org
Web site: www.dpi.org

DisAbled Women's Network (DAWN)
Canada
Web site:
www.indie.ca/dawn/index.html

Easter Seals/March of Dimes National
Council
511-90 Eglinton Ave. E.
Toronto, ON M4P 2Y3
(416) 932-8392
Fax: (416) 932-9844
TTY: (416) 932-8151
E-mail: nationalcouncil@esmodnc.org
Web site: www.esmodnc.org

Epilepsy Canada – National Office
745-1470 Peel St.
Montreal, QC H3A 1T1
(514) 845-7855
Fax: (514) 845-7866
Toll-Free: (800) 860-5499
E-mail: epilepsy@epilepsy.ca
Web site: www.epilepsy.ca/

Fragile X Research Foundation of
Canada
167 Queen St. W.
Brampton, ON L6Y 1M5
(905) 453-9366
E-mail: FXRFC@ibm.net
Web site: http://dante.med.utoronto.ca/
Fragile-X/linksto.htm

Gage Transition to Independent Living
105-100 Merton St.
Toronto, ON M4S 3G1
(416) 481-0868
Fax: (416) 481-1276
Web site: www.westpark.org

GLADNET – Global Applied Disability
Research and Information Network
P.O. Box 612, Station "B"
Ottawa, ON K1P 5P7
(613) 825-6193
Fax: (613) 825-2953
E-mail: info@gladnet.org
Web site: www.gladnet.org

Heart and Stroke Foundation of
Canada – National Office
222 Queen St., Suite 1402
Ottawa, ON K1P 5V9
(613) 569-4361
Fax: (613) 569-3278
Web site: www.hsf.ca/

Huntington Society of Canada
13 Water St. N., Suite 3
P.O. Box 1269
Cambridge, ON N1R 7G6
(519) 622-1002
Fax: (519) 622-7370
E-mail: info@hsc-ca.org
Web site: www.hsc-ca.org

International Brain Injury Association
400 Ray C. Hunt Drive, Suite 300
Charlottesville, VA 22903
(804) 243-0220
Fax: (804) 243-0333
Web site: http://ibia.vni.virginia.edu/

International Council of AIDS Service
Organizations – Central Secretariat
399 Church St.
Toronto, ON M5B 2J6
(416) 340-2437
Fax: (416) 340-8224
E-mail: icaso@web.net
Web site: www.web.org/~icaso/
webpage.html

International Society for Augmentative
and Alternative Communication
49 The Donway W., Suite 308
Toronto, ON M3C 3M9
(416) 385-0351
Fax: (416) 385-0352
E-mail: isaac_mail@mail.cepp.org
Web site: www.isaac-online.org/

Kidney Foundation of Canada,
National Office
5165 Sherbrooke St. W., Ste. 300
Montreal, QC H4A 1T6
(514) 369-4806
Fax: (514) 369-2472
Toll-Free: (800) 361-7494
E-mail: webmaster@kidney.ca
Web site: www.kidney.ca

Learning Disabilities Association of
Canada (LDAC)
200-323 Chapel St.
Ottawa, ON K1N 7Z2
(613) 238-5721
Fax: (613) 235-5391
E-mail: ldactaac@fox.nstn.ca
Web site: http://eduqueensu.ca/~lda

Lung Association of Canada – National
Office
1900 City Park Drive, Suite 508
Blair Business Park
Gloucester, ON K1J 1A3
(613) 747-6776
Fax: (613) 747-7430
Toll-Free: (888) 566-5864
Web site: www.lung.ca

Lupus Canada
P.O. Box 64034
5512 Fourth St. N.W.
Calgary, AB T2K 6J1
(403) 274-5599
Fax: (403) 274-5599
Toll-Free: (800) 661-1468
E-mail: info@lupuscanada.org
Web site: www.lupuscanada.org/

Migraine Association of Canada
356 Bloor St. E., Suite 1912
Toronto, ON M4W 3L4
(416) 920-4916
Toll-Free: (800) 663-3557
E-mail: cindy@migraine.ca
Web site: www.migraine.ca

Multiple Sclerosis Society of Canada
1000-250 Bloor St. E
Toronto, ON M4W 3P9
(416) 922-6065
Fax: (416) 922-7538
Toll-Free: (800) 268-7582
E-mail: info@mssoc.ca
Web site: www.mssoc.ca

Muscular Dystrophy Association of Canada (MDAC) – National Office
2345 Young St., Ste. 900
Toronto, ON M4P 2E5
(416) 488-0030
Fax: (416) 488-7523
Toll-Free: (800) 567-2873
Website: http://www.mdac.ca

National Aboriginal Network on Disability
www.schoolnet.ca/aboriginal/disable6/index_e.html

National Cancer Institute of Canada
10 Alcorn Ave., Suite 200
Toronto, ON M4V 3B1
(416) 961-7223
Fax: (416) 961-4189
E-mail: ncic@cancer.ca
Web site: www.cancer.ca

National Education Association of Disabled Students (NEADS)
c/o Carleton University
Room 426, 4th Level Unicenter
1125 Colonel By Drive
Ottawa, ON K1S 5B6
(613) 526-8008
Fax: (613) 520-3704
TDD: (613) 233-5963
TTY: (613) 526-8008
E-mail: neads@indie.ca
Web site: www.indie.ca/neads/

National Institute of Disability Management and Research (NIDMAR)
3699 Roger Street
Port Alberni, BC V9Y 8E3
(250) 724-4344
Fax: (250) 724- 8776
E-mail: armich@nic.bc.ca
Web site: www.nidmar.ca

North American Chronic Pain Association of Canada (NACPAC)
105-150 Central Park Drive
Brampton, ON L6T 2T9
(905) 793-5230
Fax: (905) 793-8781
Toll-Free: (800) 616-7246
Web site: www3.sympatico.ca/nacpac

Ontario Federation for Cerebral Palsy
1630 Lawrence Ave. W., Suite 104
Toronto, ON M6L 1C5
(416) 244-9686
Toll-Free: (877) 244-0899

Osteoporosis Society of Canada – National Office
P.O. Box 280, Station Q
Toronto, ON M4G 3S9
(416) 696-2663
Toll-Free: (800) 463-6842

The Parkinson Foundation of Canada
710-390 Bay St.
Toronto, ON M5H 2Y2
Toll-Free: (800) 565-3000
Web site: www.interlog.com/~
vinovich/pf/pf.html

Rick Hansen Centre
c/o University of Alberta
W1-67 Van Vliet Complex
Edmonton, AB T6G 2H9
(780) 492-9236
Fax: (780) 492-7161
Web site: www.per.Ualberta.ca/rhc/

The Roeher Institute
Kinsmen Bldg., York University
4700 Keele St.
North York, ON M3J 1P3
(416) 661-9611
Fax: (416) 661-5701
Toll-Free: (800) 856-2207
Web site: www.roeher.ca/roeher

Schizophrenia Society of Canada
814-75 The Donway W.
Don Mills, ON M3C 2E9
(416) 445-8204
Fax: (416) 445-2270
Toll-Free: (800) 809-4673
Web site: www.schizophrenia.ca

Spina Bifida and Hydrocephalus
Association of Canada
220-388 Donald St.
Winnipeg, MB R3B 2J4
(204) 925-3650
Fax: (204) 925-3654
Toll-Free: (800) 565-9488
E-mail: spinab@mts.net
Web site: www.sbhac.ca

Tetra Society of North America
27-770 Pacific Blvd. S.
Vancouver, BC V6B 5E7
(604) 688-6464
Fax: (604) 688-6463
E-mail: tetra@istar.ca
Web site: www.reachdisability.org

Tourette Syndrome Foundation of
Canada
206-194 Jarvis St.
Toronto, ON M5B 2B7
(416) 861-8398
Fax: (416) 861-2472
Toll-Free: (800) 361-3120
E-mail: tsfc.org@sympatico.ca

United Ostomy Association of Canada
Inc.
P.O. Box 46057, College Park P.O.
444 Yonge St.
Toronto, ON M5B 2L8
(416) 595-5452
Fax: (416) 595-9924
E-mail: uoacan@astral.magic.ca
http://business.atcon.com/uoacanada

The War Amps of Canada – National
Office
2827 Riverside Dr.
Ottawa, ON K1V 0C4
(613) 731-3821
Fax: (613) 731-3234
Toll-Free: (800) 465-2677
Web site: www.waramps.ca

Appendix C

Health and Disability-Related Web Sites

Able-ezine www.able-ezine.com

Abledata (database of assistive products)
www.abledata.com/index.htm

Achoo Healthcare Online (Web site index, with short descriptions)
www.achoo.com

ADA and Disability Information
www.public.iastate.edu/~sbilling/ada.html

Alzheimer's Disease www.alzheimers.org.adear

American Medical Association Home Page www.ama-assn.org

Best Information on the Internet (BIOTN) (a librarian's guide to disability resources)
www.sau.edu/cwis/internet/wild/Disabled/disindex.htm

Better Health www.betterhealth.com

Cancernet (accurate, up-to-date medical info on cancer, including a directory of experts on counselling about familial risk and genetic testing) cancernet.nci.nih.gov

Centers for Disease Control and Prevention www.cdc.gov

Clinical Pharmacology Online www.cponline.gsm.com

Cornucopia of Disability Information (CODI) (links to companies that develop or distribute adaptive computing products)
codi.buffalo.edu/graph_based/

Department of Health and Human Services (HHS)   www.hhs.gov

Disability Information Center (links to law, technology, advocacy, and Internet resources for parents, professionals, researchers, and persons with disabilities)   www.geocities.com/CapitolHill/3721/

The Disability Link Barn   www.accessunlimited.com/links.html

Family Internet (medical reference resource for diseases and other health topics)   www.familyinternet.com

The Family Village (information, resources, and communication opportunities on the Internet for persons with disabilities) www.familyvillage.wisc.edu

Food and Drug Administration   eee.fda.gov

Health Information Highway (a good source of health-related discussion groups)   www.stayhealthy.com

HealthFinder   www.healthfinder.org

HealthFinder (gateway site to find health and human services information)   www.healthfinder.gov

HealthWorld (integrates alternative health-care information) www.healthy.net

HealthyWay (lists over 8,000 linked Canadian sites) healthyway.sympatico.ca

Heart and Stroke Foundation of Canada   www.hsf.ca

HHS Administration on Aging   www.aoa.dhhs.gov/elderpage.html

HHS Health Care Financing Administration (Medicare and Medicaid information)   www.hcfa.org

Home Arts   www.homearts.com

Indian Health Service   www.ihs.gov

Information from the National Institute on Aging   www.nih.gov/nia

Integrated Network of Disability Information and Education (INDIE) (search engine and directory of resources for products, services, and information)   www.indie.ca/

Internet Medical Web Site   www.internetmedical.com

List of Online Disability Links   www.el.net/CAT/online.html

Liszt (search for discussion groups by topic)   www.liszt.com

Mayo Clinic   www.mayohealth.org

MedExplorer (information on a variety of medical subjects, including alternative medicine)   www.medexplorer.com

Medical Matrix (ranked, peer-reviewed, annotated, updated clinical medical resources, including disability links and access to numerous journals and textbooks)   www.medmatrix.org

Medicine Net   www.medicinenet.com

Mediconsult.com   www.mediconsult.com

Medline (contains an extensive collection of published medical information, including abstracts, co-ordinated by the National Library of Medicine)   igm.nlm.nih.gov/

Medscape   www.medscape.com

Medweb   www.gen.emory.edu/medweb

Merck Manual (medical reference manual written for doctors and other professionals)   www.merck.com

Mining Company — Women's Health Site
womenshealth.miningco.com/mbody.htm

National Association for Home Care   www.nahc.org

National Cancer Institute   rex.nci.nih.gov

National Institute of Health Info Page (provides a single access point to the consumer health information resources of the NIH)
www.nih.gov/health

National Institute on Life Planning homepage (dedicated to helping people with disabilities and their families plan for the future)
www.sonic.net/nilp/

Neurology Web Forum   www.mgh.harvard.edu/neurowebforum

Pharmacy Information   www.pharminfo.com

Pharmweb   www.pharmweb.net

Physicians' Choice (medical sites reviewed by physicians)
www.mdchoice.com/pcsites.htm

Quackwatch (how to avoid quackery)   www.quackwatch.com

Reuters Health   www.reutershealth.com

RxList (Internet drug list)   www.rxlist.com

Substance Abuse and Mental Health Services Administration (SAMHSA) (information about substance abuse treatment and prevention)   www.samhsa.gov

Tile.Net (search USENET newsgroups)   www.tile.net

Total Disability Bank (links to services, laws, regulations, health care, and peer support groups)   www.tdbank.com/

Treatment Findings: Agency for Health Care Policy and Research (AHCPR) (provides data to help make informed health-care decisions on specific treatment issues)   www.ahcpr.gov

TRI Online   www.idsi.net/tri/ch01-06.htm

University of Chicago Primary Care Group uhs.bsd.uchicago.edu/uhs

WebABLE! (focuses on accessibility issues on the World Wide Web) www.yuri.org/webable/

WebDoctor (helps physicians surf the Internet) www.gretmar.com/webdoctor

Wellness Web   www.wellweb.com

Yahoo Disabilities www.yahoo.com/yahoo/Society_and_Culture/Disabilities/

SEARCH ENGINES

AltaVista   www.altavista.digital.com

Excite   www.excite.com

Hotbot   www.hotbot.com

InfoSeek   www.infoseek.com

Yahoo!   www.yahoo.com

Bibliography

American Council for Headache Education, with Lynne M. Constantine and Suzanne Scott. *Migraine: The Complete Guide.* New York: Dell, 1994.

American Diabetes Association. *American Diabetes Association Complete Guide to Diabetes.* Alexandria, VA: American Diabetes Association, 1996.

American Heart Association. *American Heart Association Guide to Heart Attack: Treatment, Recovery, and Prevention.* New York: Times Books, 1996.

Bartlett, John G., and Ann K. Finkbeiner. *The Guide to Living with HIV Infection, 3d ed.* Baltimore, MD: Johns Hopkins University Press, 1996.

Bateson-Koch, Carole. *Allergies: Disease in Disguise.* Burnaby, BC: Alive Books, 1996.

Beck, Aaron T., and Gary Emery, with Ruth L. Greenberg. *Anxiety Disorders and Phobias: A Cognitive Perspective.* New York: Basic Books, 1985.

Bendall, Lisa, ed. *Directory of Disability Organozations in Canada 1998.* Toronto: Canadian Abilities Foundation, 1998.

Cameron, J. Stewart. *Kidney Failure: The Facts.* Oxford: Oxford University Press, 1996.

Cantor, Carla, with Brian A. Fallon. *Phantom Illness: Shattering the Myths of Hypochondria*. Boston: Houghton Mifflin, 1996.

Caplan, Louis R., Mark L. Dyken, and J. Donald Easton. *American Heart Association: Family Guide to Stroke*. New York: Times Books, 1994.

Carroll, David L., and Jon Dudley Dorman. *Living Well with MS: A Guide for Patient, Caregiver and Family*. New York: HarperPerennial, 1993.

Carroll, Jim, and Rick Broadhead. *Good Health Online: A Wellness Guide for Every Canadian*. Scarborough, ON: Prentice-Hall, 1997.

Catalano, Ellen Mohr, and Kimeron N. Hardin. *The Chronic Pain Control Workbook: A Step-by-Step Guide for Coping with and Overcoming Pain*. Oakland, CA: New Harbinger, 1996.

Chamberlain, Jonathon. *Fighting Cancer: A Survival Guide*. London: Headline, 1997.

Christmas, June Jackson, et al. *Every Woman's Health: The Complete Guide to Body and Mind*. New York: Simon and Schuster, 1993.

Cukier, Daniel, and Virginia McCullough. *Coping with Radiation Therapy: A Ray of Hope*. Los Angeles: Lowell House, 1996.

Dancey, Christine P., and Susan Backhouse. *A Complete Guide to Relief from Irritable Bowel Syndrome*. Phoenix: Robinson, 1997.

De Solla Price, Mark. *Living Positively in a World with HIV/AIDS: A Practical and Affirmative Guide to Refocusing and Living Your Life to the Fullest*. New York: Avon, 1995.

Dranoff, Linda Silver. *Everyone's Guide to the Law: A Handbook for Canadians*. Toronto: HarperCollins, 1997.

Eltod, Joe M. *Reversing Fibromyalgia: How to Treat and Overcome Fibromyalgia and Other Arthritis-Related Diseases*. Pleasant Grove, UT: Woodland, 1997.

Gruetzner, Howard. *Alzheimer's: A Caregiver's Guide and Sourcebook*. Toronto: John Wiley and Sons, 1992.

Harpham, Wendy Schlessel. *After Cancer: A Guide to Your New Life*. New York: HarperPerennial, 1995.

Hensel, Bruce. *Smart Medicine: How to Get the Most Out of Your Medical Checkup and Stay Healthy*. New York: Berkeley, 1996.

Irwin, John B. *Arthritis Begone!* New Canaan, CT: Keats, 1997.

Isaac, Rael Jean, and Virginia C. Armat. *Madness in the Streets: How Psychiatry and the Law Abandoned the Mentally Ill.* New York: The Free Press, 1990.

Jamison, Kay Redfield. *An Unquiet Mind: A Memoir of Moods and Madness.* New York: Knopf, 1995.

Johnson, Hillary. *Osler's Web: Inside the Labyrinth of the Chronic Fatigue Syndrome Epidemic.* Toronto: Penguin, 1996.

Klein, Bonnie Sherr. *Slow Dance: A Story of Stroke, Love and Disability.* Toronto: Vintage Canada, 1997.

LeVert, Suzanne. *When Someone You Love Has Cancer.* New York: Dell, 1995.

Long, James W. *The Essential Guide to Chronic Illness: The Active Patient's Handbook.* New York: HarperPerennial, 1997.

Love, Susan M., with Karen Lindsey. *Dr. Susan Love's Breast Book.* Don Mills, ON: Addison-Wesley, 1995.

Mabie, Margot C. J. *Bioethics and the New Medical Technology.* New York: Atheneum, 1993.

McCully, Kilmer S. *The Homocysteine Revolution.* New Canaan, CT: Keats, 1997.

McIlwain, Harris H., with Debra Fulghum Bruce. *Fibromyalgia Handbook.* New York: Owl Books, 1996.

———. *Stop Osteoporosis Now! Halting the Baby Boomers' Disease.* New York: Fireside, 1996.

McLaughlin, Chris. *Multiple Sclerosis: A Positive Approach to Living with MS.* London: Bloomsbury, 1997.

Miller, Robert H., and Christine A. Opie. *Back Pain Relief: The Ultimate Guide.* Santa Barbara, CA: Capra Press, 1997.

Moffat, Betty Clare. *The Caregiver's Companion: Words to Comfort and Inspire.* New York: Berkeley, 1997.

Morra, Marion, and Eve Potts. *The Prostate Cancer Answer Book.* New York: Avon, 1996.

Moyers, Bill. *Healing and the Mind.* Toronto: Doubleday, 1993.

Murphy, Robert F. *The Body Silent: An Anthropologist Embarks on the Most Challenging Journey of His Life: Into the World of the Disabled.* New York: Norton, 1990.

Norman, Ian J., and Sally J. Redfern. *Mental Health Care for Elderly People.* New York: Churchill Livingstone, 1997.

Notelovitz, Morris, and Diana Tonnessen. *The Essential Heart Book for Women.* New York: St. Martin's Press, 1996.

Pradell, Steven. *Winning the War Against Life-Threatening Disease.* Far Hills, NJ: New Horizon Press, 1994.

Pressman, Alan, and Herbert D. Goodman, with Karen Lane. *The Physician's Guide to Treating Arthritis, Carpal Tunnel Syndrome and Joint Conditions.* New York: Berkeley, 1997.

Reilly, Richard L. *Living with Pain: A New Approach to the Management of Chronic Pain.* Minneapolis: Deaconess Press, 1993.

Richard, Adrienne, and Joel Reiter. *Epilepsy: A New Approach.* New York: Walker and Co., 1995.

Rothman, Sheila M. *Living in the Shadow of Death: Tuberculosis and the Social Experience of Illness in America.* New York: Basic Books, 1994.

Saibil, Fred. *Crohn's Disease and Ulcerative Colitis.* Toronto: Key Porter Books, 1996.

Schlossberg, Nancy K. *Overwhelmed: Coping with Life's Ups and Downs.* San Francisco, CA: Lexington Books, 1994.

Schover, L. R. *Sexuality and Fertility After Cancer.* Toronto: Wiley, 1997.

Secunda, Victoria. *When Madness Comes Home: Help and Hope for the Children, Siblings, and Partners of the Mentally Ill.* New York: Hyperion, 1997.

Shimberg, Elaine Fantle. *Living with Tourette Syndrome.* New York: Simon and Schuster, 1995.

Thompson, John Marcus. *Arthritis.* Toronto: Key Porter Books, 1995.

Tsuang, Ming T., and Stephen V. Faraone. *Breast Cancer: A Guide for Every Woman Fighting for Life.* Oxford: Oxford University Press, 1997.

———. *The Facts Series.* Oxford: Oxford University Press, 1997.

Turkington, Carol A. *The Hearing Loss Sourcebook: A Complete Guide to Coping with Hearing Loss and Where to Get Help.* New York: Plume, 1997.

Van Bommell, Harry. *Caring for Loved Ones at Home.* Hansport, NS: Robert Pope Foundation, 1996.

Wallace, Louise M., and Christine Bundy. *Coping with Angina.* Scarborough, ON: HarperCollins, 1990.

Weisbord, Mimi. *Asthma: Breathe Again Naturally and Reclaim Your Life.* New York: St. Martin's Griffin, 1997.

Weiss, Marisa, and Ellen Weiss. *Living Beyond Breast Cancer: A Survivor's Guide for When Treatment Ends and the Rest of Your Life Begins.* New York: Times Books, 1997.

Whitehouse, Michael, and Maurice Slevin. *Cancer: The Facts.* Oxford: Oxford University Press, 1996.

Winchell, Ellen. *Coping with Limb Loss.* Garden City Park, NY: Avery Publishing Group, 1995.

Young, Pat. *The Natural Way with Arthritis and Rheumatism.* Rockport, MA: Element, 1995.

INVESTMENT BOOKS (U.S.)

Beardstown Ladies Investment Club, with Leslie Whitaker. *The Beardstown Ladies Common Sense Investment Guide: How We Beat the Stock Market — And How You Can Too.* New York: Hyperion, 1994.

Lynch, Peter, and John Rothchild. *Learn to Earn: A Beginner's Guide to the Basics of Investing and Business.* Toronto: John Wiley and Sons, 1996.

Rowland, Mary. *Best Practices for Financial Advisors.* Princeton, NJ: Bloomberg Press, 1997.

Wiegold, C. Frederic. *The Wall Street Journal Lifetime Guide to Money: Everything You Need to Know About Managing Your Finances for Every Stage of Your Life.* New York: Hyperion, 1997.

INVESTMENT BOOKS (CANADA)

Cork, David, with Susan Lighthouse. *The Pig and the Python: How to Prosper from the Aging Baby Boom.* Toronto: Stoddart Publishing, 1996.

Costello, Brian. *Taking Care of Your Money: Multi-Dimensional Investing That Works.* Toronto: ECW Press, 1997.

Croft, Richard, and Eric Kirzner. *The Beginner's Guide to Investing: A Practical Guide to Putting Your Money to Work for You.* Toronto: HarperCollins, 1997.

Janik, Carolyn, Ruth Rejnis, and Bruce McDougall. *The Complete Idiot's Guide to a Great Retirement for Canadians.* Scarborough, ON: Prentice-Hall, 1996.

Thomas Yaccato, Joanne. *Balancing Act: A Canadian Women's Financial Survival Guide.* Scarborough, ON: Prentice-Hall, 1996.

Index

Abbott, Jim, 2
access to information, 174–75
accommodations. *See* facilities
adjusting, 17–45
    barriers to, 40–45
advocacy, 98–118
    and case managers, 103, 106–7
    citizen, 102–3, 106
    designated, 102, 105
    groups, 103–4, 110–12
    legal, 103, 108–9
    local, 101–2
    national, 99–100
    personal, 261–62
    self-, 102, 104–5
    social-work sponsored, 103, 107–8
    special, 103, 109–10
    successful, 112–18
allergies, 173–74
Americans with Disabilities Act, 120
amyotrophic lateral sclerosis (ALS).
    See Lou Gehrig's disease
anger, 37, 63, 65–66, 178
assertiveness, 169–71
attitudes. *See also* stereotypes
    changing others', 27–28
    towards disabled, 7–8, 27–28
    positive, 17–20, 23–25
avoidance, dealing with, 62–63

Bell's palsy, 26
blame, attaching, 33–34
breast cancer and Internet information,
    279–83
burnout. *See* stress

caregivers, 157–80. *See also* families;
    friends; medical care; support network
    evaluating, 162, 163
    as listeners, 37
    and parents, 194–214
    respite, 140
    responsibilities, 64, 134–39
    responsibilities to, 172–73, 176–78
    selecting, 163–69
    and stress, 138–40, 181–93
cerebral palsy, 7, 27–28, 46
chart, personnel, 179
Charter of Rights and Freedoms
    (Canadian), 120
children comprehending disability,
    52–53
computers, 94–95, 137, 275–86
    and breast cancer information,
    279–83
    and fibromyalgia information,
    283–84
    and the Internet, 277–86
    and misinformation, 276–77

offers of payment, 262–64, 267–68
premium return, 238
premium waiver, 239
retirement rider, 239
settlements, 268–70
sickness wording, 240
supplementary disability, 240
underwriting, 238
Internet. *See* computers
isolation, 63–64, 117–18, 155

Klein, Bonnie Sherr, 171–72
Klippel-Trenaunay-Weber syndrome,
127–28

labels. *See* stereotypes
legal
action, 33–34, 108–9, 116, 119–30,
168
problems, 122–28
protection, 255–60
settlements, 129
living will, 175–76
Lou Gehrig's disease, 2, 21–22, 53

Martin, Casey, 127–28
Medic Alert, 173–74
medical care, 157–80. *See also*
caregivers
medical claims, 260–68
medical options, 171–72
mental illness, 32–33
Merrick, John, 23
multiple sclerosis, 96, 152–53

negative thinking, 8
negligence, 125–26

opinions, second, 160–61
options, choosing, 35, 171–72. *See
also* treatment
ostomy, 17–18
overindulgence, dealing with, 59–60

paralysis, 31
parents
and accommodation choices,

198–204
in caregiver's home, 199, 203–7
caregiving for, 194–214
and independent living, 202–3,
207–11
and institutional living, 211–14
resolving differences with, 200–202
responsibility to, 197–98
patronization. *See* condescension
personal-injury lawyer, 261–62
pity, dealing with, 59–60
planning, 10, 52, 57, 112–13, 157–69,
197. *See also* protection plan
financial, 249–53
power of attorney, 171, 175–76
for personal care, 258–59
for property, 255–57
privacy, 54, 64
programs, custom-designed, 153–55
protection plan
building, 231–54
components, 232–42
importance of, 217–30

quadriplegia, 1, 43–44, 90, 150
and Internet information, 284–85

reasonable (definition), 122
records, keeping, 173
Reeve, Christopher, 1, 90
research projects, participating in, 168
residence. *See* housing options
resources, 9. *See also* planning
respite care, 140
responsibility, taking, 35. *See also*
attitudes, positive
Roosevelt, Franklin Delano, 2

schizophrenia, 32–33
scleroderma, 36
self-education. *See* planning
self-image, 20–28
self-isolation, 38–39
service clubs, 145–46
services, public, 121
settlement
insurance, 268–70